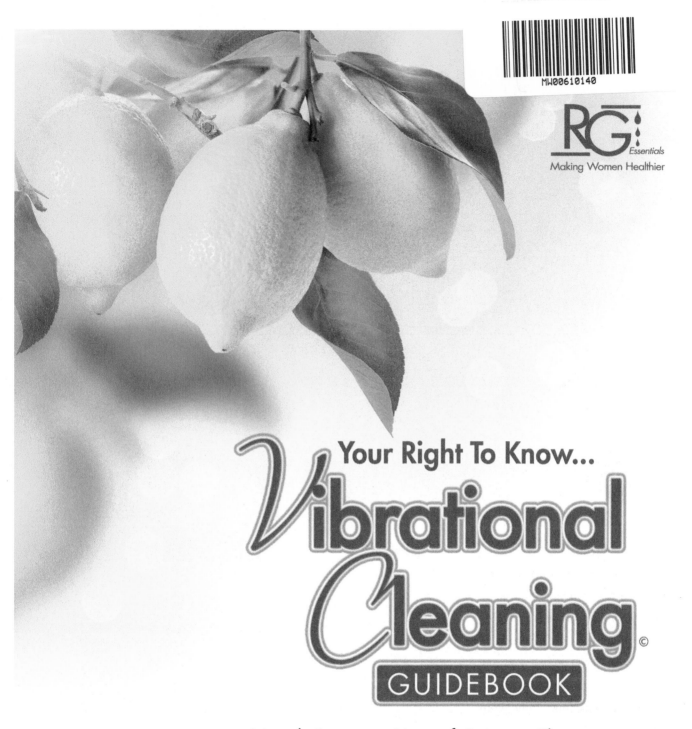

RG Essentials
Making Women Healthier

Your Right To Know...

Vibrational Cleaning GUIDEBOOK ©

Novel, Dynamic Uses of Genuine Therapeutic
Essential Oils that can change your life

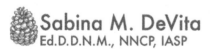

Sabina M. DeVita
Ed.D.D.N.M., NNCP, IASP

Over 100 Food Preparations & Home-office Cleaning
Tips that also help Supercharge your brain!

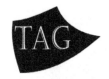

Available From:

Wellness Institute of Living and Learning

7700 Hurontario St., Suite 408

Brampton, ON Canada L6Y 4M3

(905) 451-4475

info@devitawellness.com

info@energywellnessstudies.com

ISBN: 978-1-59930-435-9

Important Notice

The author makes no claims nor is rendering professional advice or service to the individual reader. The information in this book is intended for educational purposes only. It should not replace the recommendations or advice provided by your physician.

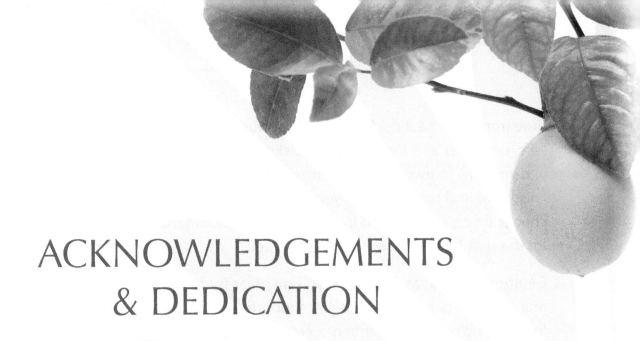

ACKNOWLEDGEMENTS & DEDICATION

I dedicate this follow-up book entitled "Your Right To Know - Vibrational Cleaning Guidebook" to my creator, the God-head, the Infinite source for all of my inspiration, creative ideas and the sustaining energy of light to keep me on my path. I also dedicate this book to humanity- my Light Family **for Our Spiritual Evolution to expand in peace, in love and in connection to our Infinite Source. A very special thank you to these individuals:**

D. Gary Young- I specifically thank you, Gary Young for your ingenuity, dedication, your love, your commitment & truthfulness in growing, distilling and producing the world's best in 'edible' genuine, God-preserved essential oils for humanity's awakening, healing and transformation on our planet on all levels- body, mind & spirit. I appreciate all that you do and have created for us Gary. I have witnessed you working in the fields, driving the semi-truck, cutting the trees, reforesting, planting, your sustainable farming practices and seeing your new inventions- like the Highland Flats distillery, your creative design of the world's first computerized stainless steel distillery to help shift the consciousness for humanity. I honor and love you and I appreciate all your hard work to maintain God's purity of Light in these special 'bottles of Light'. I value and hold dearly our unique friendship and connection in serving the human race. Without you I would not be involved in doing what I have been doing with the essential oils nor in writing this book. I feel truly blessed and treasure the gift of the essential oils that you have ushered in to our current times while integrating the knowledge of the ancient past to our modern scientific advances today.

Mary Young- I thank you Mary for being so willing and so present in furthering the 'needed awakening' to who we truly are in our current world. Your feedback has further inspired me ... that this guidebook has finally materialized. Thank you for taking the time from your hectic schedule as the Young Living executive Vice President, mother, wife, presenter and the myriads of tasks you do, to read my Vibrational Cleaning book and write my foreword. I appreciate your special friendship, love and your care for us all. I also love and honor all that you do to preserve the integrity of these genuine, 100% chemical free, essential oils in order to have true, organically grown, therapeutic quality for the shift in consciousness on our planet.

Geoffrey my husband - I thank you my dear for supporting me in my ventures in so many ways and particularly, being supportive during my late night writing. Thanks too for enjoying my experimenting 'scentsably' in our home. I love you for who you are.

To my friends, I thank you all for your positive feedback and encouragement. I bless you as you have blessed and enriched my life. I thank those in my family who have also encouraged and supported me on my quest for truth and in my teachings.

To all of you who are reading this book, May Great Spirit bless you, as you assist in truly 'greening' the planet in mind, body and heart-soul. Mother Earth certainly thanks you too.

LEARN REAL GREEN MAKEOVERS FOR:

All Round Green Home Scents, Green Kitchen scents, Bathroom scents,

Laundry scents, Deodorant scents, Insect- pest Scents...... Well- it makes a lot of common 'Scents' when using pure, genuine essential oils!

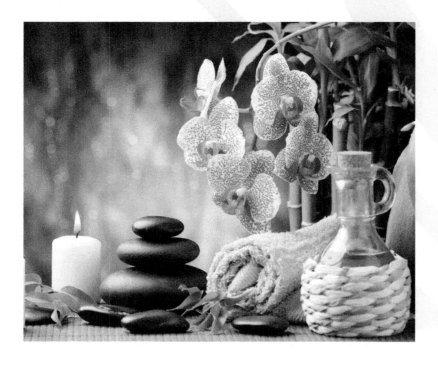

Vibrational Cleaning is a Common 'Scents' Way of green cleaning that is novel in utilizing current research in aromas and the brain as well as the disinfecting powers of genuine therapeutic essential oils. This way of cleansing will help to activate your pineal and supercharge your brain capabilities all while cleaning.

Read my first book on "Vibrational Cleaning" if you haven't already, for more details about what the toxic cleaning household chemicals do to the pineal gland! Every home or office is cleaned at some point whoever is responsible --- so you might as well clean and help to heal the people in your environments at the same time.

YOUR RIGHT TO KNOW - VIBRATIONAL CLEANING GUIDEBOOK ©
"Real Green Essentials: Making Women Healthier"

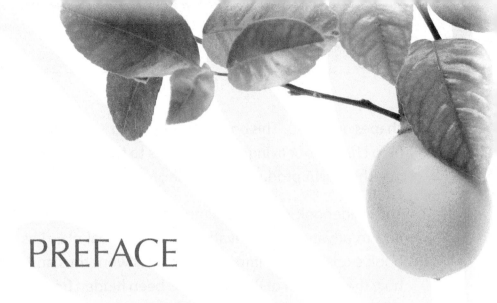

PREFACE

When a number of readers gave me an overwhelming amount of positive feedback and acknowledgement for my Vibrational Cleaning book in how it made a significant difference in changing their lives, I knew that it was time to write a follow-up recipe 'greening' guidebook. When Mary Young, Executive Vice President of Young Living Company, had also expressed her encouragement for me to create a menu-type guidebook, after reading my first book and writing a foreword for it, I knew that it was time to follow through in writing this book. So here it is the ***"Your Right To Know.. Vibrational Cleaning Guidebook – Novel, Dynamic Uses of Genuine Therapeutic Essential Oils that can change your life"*** that you now have in your hands as you are reading this.

Having safe, clean and healing environments has become even more important today due to the onslaught of environmental pollutants, chemicals and the global epidemics of the antibiotic-resistant bacteria's also known as the **superbugs.** Environmental toxins can be found everywhere in what we eat, drink, breathe, wash and clean with. You may not be aware of these toxins, but they are impacting you in how you think, feel and behave – compromising your immune system and specifically targeting your brain. So if you desire to be healthy today, it is a must in being educated on the toxic chemical overload and what to do in making significant healthy life-style changes! We're discovering that too many chronic conditions, like type 2 diabetes, cardiovascular disease, cancer, lymphoma and obesity, are now being linked directly to environmental toxins in your body. Furthermore, with the advances in quantum physics and quantum biology, we now know that the role of these environmental toxins (be it food toxins, heavy metals, stress, our words etc) is what shapes our DNA- a new field in genetics, as discovered by Dr. Bruce Lipton, called "Epi-genetics" (how our environment dictates &

shapes our DNA). This book, "Your Right To Know - Vibrational Cleaning Guidebook" is to help change our living environments to healthy, vibrant clean ones that will help shape healthier DNA producing healthier, happier lives.

This guidebook is meant to simplify many of the formulas offered in 'Vibrational Cleaning" and to advance the activation of your pineal gland as well at the same time. My first book explained the importance of this wondrous and super powered gland, outlining how the function of the pineal has been hidden from us for thousands of years and how chemical toxins block and calcify it. I encourage you to read this book in its entirety to understand the 'secrets' kept from humanity. With this guidebook, I show a unique, simple, all-organic and amazingly powerful vibrational plant-based *household cleaning method* that helps to rid the chemical toxins and furthermore help you to activate your *intuitive center- your pineal gland at the same time*.

Now you can reduce and even eliminate the use of dangerous chemicals and neuro toxins found in your typical household and personal care products that you currently buy. In unison, we can all make a major difference to the air we breathe, the food we eat and the water we drink by what our pocketbook supports.

I thank this one reader who wrote a most profound and succinct endorsement about my first book. She found it to be so helpful that she wanted others to know as well. "Cleaning your home and opening up your intuitive sense all at once? This amazing book presents new and life-altering information clearly and logically. The most profound shifts often come from making the simplest changes." Helping families make the simplest changes was certainly one of my goals in my first book and so it is with this guidebook as well. This way our cleaning routines can become habitual.

Mary Young also stated in her Foreword to my first book: "*Vibrational Cleaning* is one of the most valuable books anyone can read who is looking for answers and solutions to living in our polluted and toxic world… See the results of greater health and wellness, and most of all, life-giving freedom."

This guidebook, especially for busy people, will show you many simple and life-supporting life-style benefits in truly going Green. Take a few moments each day to integrate the many 'greening' tips and you'll be pleased that you have. Your home 'scents' will help to revitalize you, awaken you, protect you from infections including the Superbugs, as well as keep your home/office safe, healthy and clean- the 'Real Green' Way!

AUTHOR'S SPECIAL NOTE:

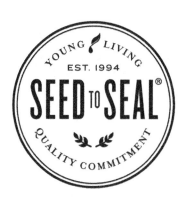

I have chosen Young Living essential oils Company as my primary and only choice in using or recommending essential oils due to their authenticity and guarantee that they are pure, 100% chemical free, organically grown by sustainable and ecological farming practices. Young Living owns & operates their own farms now in 11 countries and upholds the prominent seal of **"Seed to Seal'** distinction in the aromatherapy industry.

Obviously, if you can find the same standard of edible and impeccable clean, environmental sustainable essential oils then by all means, go ahead, they will be a great asset to you. There are a very few companies that can meet this challenge. Ask your company pertinent questions in its production in all areas from seed to cultivation, growth and distillation practices and verify their information. Otherwise you will purchase essential oils that will not offer you all the marvellous benefits outlined in this guidebook.

Since I have had the opportunity to visit and work on a few of the Young Living farms and have seen firsthand what is involved with producing high quality Genuine, food-grade therapeutic essential oils, along with the documentation in their rigorous testing, I feel confident to suggest using these **true** 'Eco- Green' Young Living essential oils to you. Let us enjoy these unadulterated treasured gifts from Mother Nature in all that she offers us. As author *Rudolf Steiner* once said:

"Matter is the most spiritual in the perfume of plants." May you bless your presence & your environments with the true 'spirits' from these precious perfumes of plants - the Nature Spirits.

9

TABLE OF CONTENTS

REAL GREEN CLEAN THE VIBRATIONAL WAY

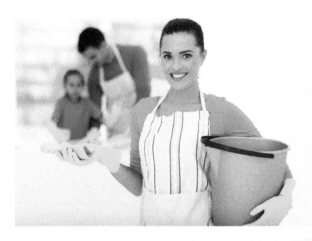

Here are your handy tips to really "green" clean your home's dirtiest rooms with ease and comfort – that will leave your home sparkling, refreshing, non-toxic and safe in no time!

House cleaning is most often not viewed as a pleasant task- nor does it need to be viewed as tedious or strenuous or for that matter time consuming.

Now you can prepare for a most delightful, 'aromatizing' experience that will leave your senses heightened while soothed. Spiritual awakening or enlightenment can also happen anywhere and at anytime, even while cleaning. You can practice a unique 'being in the moment' experience or 'mindfulness' as you surround yourself with the uplifting aromas and focus 'being' in the 'NOW'.

Plan ahead and follow these tips listed in this guidebook to create a peace-filled, harmonious, 'heavenly' space to awaken your mind's eye, open to your Infinite Potential and retain your memory all while *'vibrationally'* cleaning.

**Your eco-green guide to *Vibrational Cleaning*
Kitchen Scents First**

CHAPTER 1

Greening your Kitchen
The Importance of Hygiene & Safety

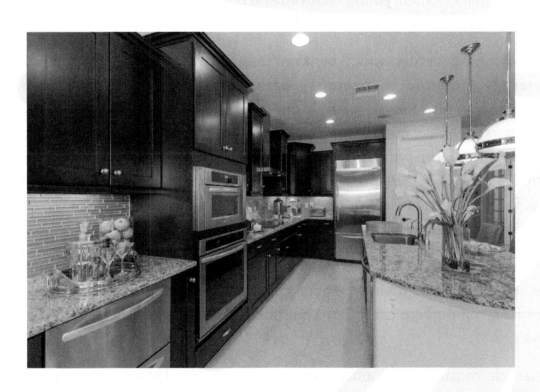

*"All the Flowers of all the tomorrows
are in the seeds of today"*

Indian Proverb

The kitchen is the most significant area in a home to be concerned about in regards to hygiene and safety. This is where food is prepared and often eaten. Hygiene, disinfecting, food protection and food preservation are critical for good health. In my "Vibrational cleaning" book, I presented the statistics of how over _76 million cases of food poisoning takes place every year,_ with 80 percent of them being caused at home. It is a _very real threat that can leave a family devastated:_ According to the Centres for Disease Control and Prevention (CDC), every year, **_one in six_** Americans gets sick after eating contaminated foods. Some of these symptoms can manifest as upset stomach, abdominal cramps, diarrhea and/or vomiting which may not be life-threatening; but for some it is! Approximately, 128,000 are hospitalized and about 3,000 people die from foodborne diseases. It is estimated that about **_11 million Canadians experience food poisoning each year_** with the greatest risk for food poisoning being seniors, pregnant women, **young children and babies** and people with chronic medical conditions (e.g., diabetes, AIDS, liver disease).

Food poisoning occurs when contaminated foods or water (bacterial toxins (substances produced by bacteria), parasites, or viruses, are ingested. Food poisoning can also occur when non-infectious poisons (such as poisonous mushrooms) or heavy metals (such as lead or mercury) find their way into people's digestive tracts. The symptoms common to all food poisoning are nausea, vomiting, abdominal cramps and diarrhea. Bacterial toxins tend to cause these symptoms as well as fever and headache. Symptoms can start within hours to days after eating the contaminated food and last from a day to a week.

More serious symptoms are ones that are caused by many non-infectious poisons (not caused by bacteria and their toxins, viruses, etc) that affect the central nervous system and cause symptoms typical of nerve poisons that cause weakness, skin rashes, pain or paralysis.

For example, mushroom poisoning also attacks the central nervous system. Symptoms such as shrunken eye pupils, tears, salivation or frothing at the mouth, sweating, vertigo, confusion, coma, and sometimes seizures can appear within 2 hours of eating a poisonous mushroom. Insecticides based on organophosphates can cause very similar symptoms. These food-borne & pesticide issues are a global problem that take place in any country.

Food poisoning caused by the bacteria _Listeria_ can cause problems for unborn babies and _E. coli_ infection can cause problems with the kidneys. Other complications can include arthritis and bleeding problems. Non-infectious food poisoning can occasionally lead to permanent nervous system problems and even death. The CDC reports that the leading causes of foodborne deaths were Nontyphoidal _Salmonella_, _Toxoplasma_, _Listeria_ and Norovirus.

Due to the seriousness of food poisoning alone, I have added more research for you as to the life-saving benefits that organic, pure; food-grade essential oils will offer you and your family. Most people are just unaware of what essential oils offer and resort to products like chlorine bleach which is toxic and causes other environmental issues. (See 'Vibrational Cleaning' book) You can do much to prevent food poisoning in your own kitchen with the understanding that **many essential oils are powerful disinfectants and antiseptics and will ward off salmonella, _E. coli_ and other pathogens, where other most used chemical agents won't.**

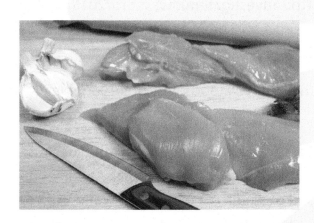

According to Environmental Working Group's latest March 2013 report, superbugs are on the rise—and they're in supermarkets!. Tests of **ground raw turkey conducted in 2006 found that 82 percent of _E. coli_ bacteria (responsible for 6 million infections a year) were antibiotic-resistant.**[1] In 2011, federal scientists determined that **74 percent of the salmonella bacteria on raw chicken were antibiotic-resistant, up from less than 50 percent in 2002.**

Every Year, according to the Centres for Disease Control and Prevention (CDC), salmonella enterica bacterium causes about 1.2 million illnesses in the United States. (http://www.cdc.gov/salmonella) Salmonella accounts for 23,000 hospitalizations and 450 deaths a year. Most persons infected with _Salmonella_ develop diarrhea, fever, and abdominal cramps 12 to 72 hours after infection that usually lasts four to seven days. Children are the most likely to become infected with salmonella. CDC reports that the rate of _diagnosed infections in children less than five years old_ is higher than the rate in all other persons. Young children are particularly at high risk for foodborne illnesses- so parents need to become aware of this and use many preventive measures. Many natural guidelines are outlined for you in this book.

With 42 years of laboratory-confirmed surveillance, the CDC data on **30 Salmonella serotypes** have been identified. The most common foods that harbor salmonella are beef, poultry, milk and eggs but are also found in **fruits, vegetables and nuts.**

Another example of a rare food that was most recently identified by the CDC as a cause of a salmonella outbreak (July 14, 2014, a total of 25 persons were infected with salmonella reported from 14 states) was organic sprouted Chia powder! This isn't a food that most would associate with Salmonella but it does show how any food can become infected.

Salmonella –E-coli in Ground Beef

Today, all beef that is tested for E. coli is also tested for salmonella, but if ground beef tests positive for salmonella, it can still enter the food chain. The bacteria are often the result of cross-contamination with raw foods, or from contamination from humans, animals, birds or reptiles. Simply, any food processing plant that isn't careful about cross-contamination is essentially at risk. (http://investigatemidwest.org/2013/09/19/food-safety-officials-tweak-salmonella-testing-process) The food is only recalled if it's linked to human illness.

According to Foods Safety government: (http://www.foodsafety.gov/blog/sneaky_salmonella.html)

"it gets into food through the poop of animals, such as cows, birds, and mice. Because the natural home for *Salmonella* bacteria is in the gut of these animals, their poop becomes a carrier of the germ if it gets into food or water. For example, if water used to irrigate a field has animal poop in it, the water can contaminate the food growing in the field." Contamination can also occur where food is being made by a tainted ingredient that can get on equipment and spread.

CHICKEN

In 2013, chickens were the largest known source of salmonella, as stated above at 74% with outbreaks connected to 615 different reported salmonella infections. But it's not only occurring in meat products. Here are a few other foods that have been identified.

FREEZE-DRIED FRUIT

Early in 2014, 59,780 cases of freeze-dried Kirkland Signature Real Sliced Fruit produced exclusively for Costco Wholesale Stores were recalled because of potential salmonella contamination. (http://www.foodsafetynews.com/2014/03/kirkland-signature-sliced-fruit-recalled-from-costco-for-potential-salmonella/#.Uz7wYK2Syoo)

Packaged fruit can contain salmonella if the factory in which it was processed was contaminated or if the fruit in question came into contact with the bacteria before it was packaged.

Other foods that were found to be contaminated with salmonella, highlights the fact that you can't always avoid salmonella just by avoiding raw meats. It was found (very rare) in *organic basil, peanut butter and Raw Cashew Cheese.* When it comes to organic basil- the maxim is simple: know your grower or your producer!

As the CDC warns: Don't wash meat, poultry and eggs! This can actually spread *Salmonella* to other foods.

WHAT TO DO? ESSENTIAL OIL RESEARCH

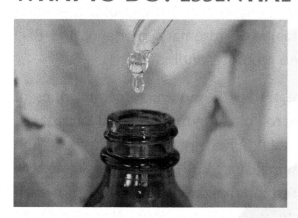

It sounds scary perhaps in what is happening to these types of food contaminations but **protecting** yourself is easy with **essential oils** as they have been proven to be extremely valuable in food preservation and food safety. Studies have been conducted worldwide in various countries as to the effectiveness of essential oils as anti-bacterial and anti-pathogenic agents.

For the past decade, a series of studies in food microbiology have been testing the efficacy of essential oils for food storage purposes as well as food preservation. These studies were conducted at the Université du Québec's Research Laboratories in Sciences Applied to Food, and were published in the peer-reviewed *Journal of Agricultural and Food Chemistry* in 2004 and 2005.

One such study applied an essential oils mix containing **oregano oil** on beef. Results showed that **the use of film containing** essential oils significantly reduced the growth of pathogenic bacteria, **including _E. coli,_ as compared to meat that was non-treated.** The researchers concluded: "The application of bioactive films on meat surfaces … showed that film containing oregano oil was the most effective against both bacteria's."[1]

In another study, the authors assert that essential oils and their components are active against a wide variety of microorganisms, including pathogenic Gram-negative bacteria. Several oils were tested for efficacy with the _Pseudomonas putida_ strain. Seven essential oils were shown to have strong antimicrobial activity against _P. putida,_ while ten other oils also showed a high antimicrobial activity at a different dilution rate.[2]

The Center for Food Safety, University of Arkansas, conducted a study against three strains of _E. coli_ 157:H7 using a variety of **_orange essential oil._** The June 2012 study concluded that orange oil can be used against E-coli: "the research reported here indicates that some of these oils may be used as surface applications during cold temperatures to inhibit the food borne pathogen _E. coli_ 0157:H7."

A French study also analyzed the effects of certain essential oil constituents in broiler chickens, that can be used as an **alternative antibiotic**- they focused on **rosemary**, **oregano** and a commercial blend of **cinnamaldehyde** and **1,8 cineole**. The study reported that "In general, essential oils contained in rosemary, oregano, and BEO [blended essential oils] can substitute for growth promoter antibiotics."

Food scientists at the University of Delaware tested the antimicrobial activities of essential oil constituent's **thymol** and **carvacrol** plus **thyme** essential oil against Salmonella on grape tomatoes. What did they find? Here is their conclusion: "The uses of these antimicrobial agents achieved significant log reductions of Salmonella on inoculated grape tomatoes and decreased dramatically the risk of potential transmission of pathogens from tomatoes to washing solutions. None of these antimicrobial agents decreased the total phenolic and ascorbic acid content, nor did any of them change the color and pH values or affect the taste, aroma, or visual quality of grape tomatoes. Therefore, 0.4 mg/ml thymol has great potential to be an alternative to chlorine-based washing solution for fresh produce."[15]

FRESH PRODUCE OR TOXIC GREENS: MORE RESEARCH

Vegetables account for about one-third of all cases of food poisoning in the US, and the worst offenders are the leafy greens, such as ***spinach, lettuce and kale.*** They are the highest-risk producers as these vegetables grow close to the ground and are easily contaminated from irrigation water and livestock runoff. Leafy greens also have shapes and textures that make them harder to clean than other types of produce.

Those who enjoy the convenience of packaged salads will be relieved to know researchers in Spain tested **oregano** essential oil and **citral**, found in **lemongrass, petitgrain, lime, lemon, and orange essential oils,** in packaging film against *Escherichia coli, Salmonella enterica* and *Listeria monocytogenes*. The study investigated the essential oil and constituent both "in vitro" [in an artificial environment like a test tube] and also on the food itself. The results were very promising: they showed that the "antimicrobial activity reduced spoilage flora on the salad as well as inhibited the growth of pathogens in contaminated salads. This effect was greater against Gram-negative bacteria. Sensory studies showed that the package that was most effective and most accepted by customers was the one containing 5% oregano essential oil."[16]

In another study (published in 2007) conducted at the Canadian Irradiation Center Research Laboratory in Sciences Applied to Food, INRS-Institut Armand-Frappier, Université du Québec, the researchers Mounia Oussalah, Stéphane Caillet, Linda Saucier, & Monique Lacroix set out to test the inhibitory effects of essential oils on the growth of four specific pathogenic bacteria. Twenty eight essential oils were evaluated for their antibacterial properties, specifically against four pathogenic bacteria (*Escherichia coli O157:H7, Listeria monocytogenes 2812 1/2a, Salmonella Typhimurium SL 1344 and Staphylococcus aureus*).

Results showed that the most active essential oils against the bacteria tested were Corydothymus capitatus, (**Spanish origanum**) Cinnamomum cassia, (**Cassia**) Origanum heracleoticum, (**Greek Oregano**), Satureja montana,(**Mountain Savory)** **and** Cinnamomum verum (**True Cinnamon bark**). Corydothymus capitatus was the most active. The authors concluded that '**As food preservatives, volatile oils may have their greatest potential use.'** (2)

Another study by Penalver P, Huerta B, Borge C, et al researched the antimicrobial activity *of essential oils of Cory*dothymus capitatus (**Spanish origanum**), Satureja montana, (**Mountain Savory)** Thymus mastichina (**Spanish Origanum majorana**),

"The essential oil that showed the highest antimicrobial activity against the four strains of *Salmonella* was *Origanum vulgare* (**Oregano**) followed by *Thymus zygis* (**Thyme**), *Thymus mastichina* (**Wild Marjoram, Sweet Marjoram**) which inhibited all the microorganisms at the highest concentration, while the rest of the essential oils showed highly variable results.

The authors concluded that the results of this work confirmed the antimicrobial activity of some essential oils, as well as their potential application in the treatment and prevention of poultry and pig diseases caused by salmonella. (3)

Another more recent study in the *Journal of Food Science*, published by the Institute of Food Technologists (IFT), July 2014, found that essential oils may be able to be used as **_food preservatives in packaging to help extend the shelf-life_** of food products. (4)

The bread of life has taken on a new 'aroma' as scientists tap into food preservation using essential oils. Another 2014 study from ACS *Journal of Agricultural and Food Chemistry* reports the development of new edible films containing oils from **_clove and oregano_** that preserve bread longer than commercial additives. A team of scientists decided to test how well different edible films with **clove and oregano** essential oils could maintain bread's freshness in comparison to a commercial antimicrobial agent.

The scientists placed preservative –free bread slices in plastic bags with or without essential oil-infused edible films. Some slices were preserved with a commercial preservative containing calcium propionate. The results after 10 days showed that the commercial additive lost its effectiveness, but the edible films made with small droplets of the two essential oils continued to slow mold growth. [5]

All these studies point out significant findings as to the strong antimicrobial activity of essential oils and how they can be applied in the prevention of foodborne illnesses, food safety, disinfectants, storage and preservation. Essential oils are booming in popularity amongst scientists today as more people are becoming aware of the toxic chemicals found in all aspects of their lives: from food to cleaners. More consumers are seeking for more alternatives to replace their synthetic cleaning products, toxic personal care items, anti-mosquito sprays and even their medicines. This guidebook is directly addressing these environmental and health issues.

24

ANOTHER PATHOGEN ON THE RISE: CAMPYLOBACTER

Another infectious pathogen and one of the most common causes of diarrheal illness in the United States is Campylobacteriosis which is a disease caused by a spiral –shaped bacteria of the genus *Campylobacter*. Centers for Disease & Control report that most people who become ill with Campylobacteriosis experience diarrhea which may be bloody accompanied by nausea & vomiting, cramping, abdominal pain and fever within two to five days after exposure to the organism. The illness typically affects those with compromised immune systems and can last about a week. In more severe cases, the infection can cause a serious life-threatening infection. CDC reports that **Campylobacter Outbreaks have been on the rise since 2009 with many that go unreported. It is estimated to affect over 1.3 million persons every year**.

Contamination or infection can occur ***from even one drop of juice from raw chicken meat*** which can have enough *Campylobacter* in it to infect a person! It's easy to do on just an *unwashed cutting board* after poultry meat was cut on it- as *Campylobacter* organisms can infect other foods that are cut on the same cutting board.

How to wash your cutting board? There are safe and reliable ways in using essential oils to clean your cutting board s which are detailed in chapter 2. Presented below is another study that specifically shows an additional benefit in the effectiveness of applying essential oils for campylobacter. Hence, essential oils become a wise choice to use on your cutting boards, your knives and your countertops, literally using the oils anywhere in your kitchen and on your food.

A SAFE NATURAL SOLUTION

In this study, the researchers wanted to investigate the effectiveness of oils and vapours of **lemon** (Citrus limon), **sweet orange** (Citrus sinensis) and **bergamot** (Citrus bergamia) and their components against a number of common foodborne pathogens that included **E.coli** and **Campylobacter, Listeria monocytogenes, Bacillus cereus and Staphylococcus aureus in vitro and in food systems.**

Bergamot was found to be the most effective of the oils and linalool the most effective anti-bacterial component. The researchers conclude that the results suggest the possibility that citrus EOs, particularly bergamot, could be used as a way of combating the growth of common causes of food poisoning. (5)

These studies clearly demonstrate how essential oils have real use as natural protectors of our food and health. The authors point out that essential oils have 'long served as flavoring agents in food and beverages, and due to their versatile content of antimicrobial compounds, they possess potential as natural agents for food preservation'.

David Gutierrez, staff writer for **Natural News (Aug. 2014)** writes about another more recent study that was conducted by researchers from Washington State University and was published in the journal *Food Control* in December 2014. They found that the essential oil of **cinnamon** is a potent antibacterial agent that may be useful as a natural method for preventing the spread of foodborne illness.

The researchers tested the essential oil against the top six strains of a variety of *Escherichia coli* (*E. coli*) bacteria known as Shiga toxin-producing *E. coli*, or non-O157 STEC. They found that just **10 drops of cinnamon essential oil in a liter of water** were able to kill all six strains of non-O157 STEC **within 24 hours**.

Since the U.S. Department of Agriculture Food Safety and Inspection Service has a "zero tolerance" policy for any of these 6 strains found in any of the food products, this finding is another major breakthrough in food preservation. Lina Sheng one of the researchers commented that: "The oil can be incorporated into films and coatings for packaging both meat and fresh produce," ….. It can also be added into the washing step of meat, fruits or vegetables to eliminate microorganisms."

There has been a growing concern over the health effects of chemical preservatives and other food additives which have led to a growing market for natural alternatives. This has spurred many scientists to research natural solutions. David Gutierrez also points out other very exciting studies being conducted world-wide in his article.

Scientists in a 2006 study at Spain's University of Extremadura found that essential oils of **rosemary and sage** were actually more effective at preventing meat spoilage than either BHA or BHT. Another study, in 2008, that was conducted by Portuguese researchers and published in the journal *Innovative Food Science and Emerging Technologies* found that olive and grape extracts (byproducts of olive oil and wine making) were also more effective preservatives than pure chemical antioxidants. (6)

COMMON "SCENTS' HYGIENE PRACTICES

Below are some 'scents-able' & **life-saving** ways in *how you can minimize your risk for foodborne illnesses …and feel healthy as well.*

The number 1 practice for any kitchen is hygiene- basic cleaning practices. The CDC outlines the importance of these 5 basic ways to clean (I have added essential oils rather than using chlorine for cleaning sinks or countertops) as bacteria can spread throughout the kitchen via the hands, cutting boards, utensils, counter tops and food. To reduce bacterial infections remember:

Wash your hands with warm water and **Thieves soap** for at least 20 seconds before and after handling food and after using the bathroom, changing diapers and/or handling pets.

Wash your cutting boards, dishes, utensils, and counter tops with hot soapy water using **Thieves household cleaner** (also spray **Thieves or lemon, orange, or oregano** oil after preparing each food item and before you go on to the next food).

Consider using paper towels to clean up kitchen surfaces. If you use cloth towels wash them often in the hot cycle of your washing machine- by adding 15 drops or more of **Thieves, Melaleuca, Lemon or Thyme** oil to the wash.

Rinse fresh fruits and vegetables under running cold tap water, including those with skins and rinds that are not eaten- soak produce in water /essential oil combination. See Soaking Fruits and Vegetables in Chapter 2.

Rub firm-skin fruits and vegetables under running cold tap water or scrub with a clean vegetable brush dipped in a solution of **citrus oils** and water while rinsing with running tap water.

CHART OF FOOD- BORNE BACTERIA
– ESSENTIAL OIL SOLUTIONS

Types of bacteria	Essential oils studied for effectiveness
E-Coli & *Pseudomonas putida* strain	Oregano oil
E. coli 157:H7 (3 strains)	Orange oil
Salmonella (various strains)	oregano & thyme essential oils
Escherichia coli, Salmonella enterica and *Listeria monocytogenes.*	Oregano, lemongrass, petitgrain, lime, lemon, and orange essential oils
Chicken antibiotic	Rosemary, oregano, and a commercial blend of cinnamaldehyde and 1,8 cineole.
Escherichia coli O157:H7, Listeria monocytogenes 2812 1/2a, Salmonella Typhimurium SL 1344 and Staphylococcus aureus	Corydothymus capitatus (Spanish origanum) Cinnamomum cassia, (Chinese cassia or Chinese cinnamon), Origanum heracleoticum (Greek oregano), Satureja montana, (Mountain Savory) and Cinnamomum verum (Ceylon cinnamon or True cinnamon)
Campylobacter, E.coli, Listeria monocyto-genes, Bacillus cereus and Staphylococcus aureus in vitro and in food systems.	Lemon (Citrus limon), sweet orange (Citrus sinensis), and bergamot
Shiga toxin-producing *E. coli*, or non-O157 STEC	Cinnamon oil

CHAPTER 2

Vibrational Cleaning Kitchen Guidelines

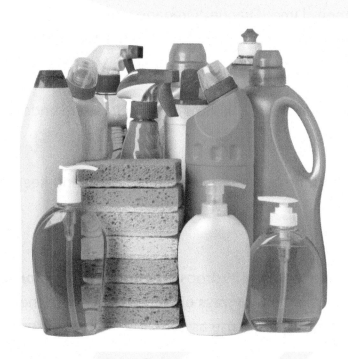

YOUR HOUSEHOLD GREEN SCENTS- UTENSILS

Use common 'scents' to go green, energetically attune your space and activate your mind's eye!

All you need: Pail, sponges, baking soda, vinegar, Borax, apple cider vinegar, Spritzer bottles and your YL Essential oils!

HOW TO MAKE YOUR OWN REAL GREEN CLEANERS
PREPARING YOUR SPRITZER BOTTLES BEFOREHAND

1. Drop 5-8 drops of one of the essential oils listed below per 8 ounce size bottle (more oil for bigger spray bottles). It is wise to prepare at least 6 different bottles for the kitchen and another 3 for other areas in the home, such as your laundry room and bathroom.

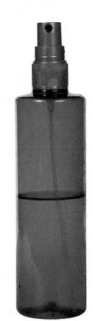

2. Then fill the bottle with water and shake before using.
Suggested oils: Lemon, Lime, Bergamot, Citrus Fresh, Lemongrass, Oregano, Thyme, Marjoram, Palmarosa, Orange, Melrose, Thieves or Purification (many to choose from)
I usually have Lemon, Lime, Orange, Oregano and Thieves bottles on my own kitchen countertop, ready to use for food and kitchen sanitation.

Another 3 bottles of Purification, Palmarosa and Melrose are under the sink ready to use elsewhere in the home.

I also prepare my scouring powder beforehand as well and keep my mixture in a jar ready to use.

Scouring Powder
- To one cup of baking soda, add 20 drops of **Lemon, Purification, Lavender, Cypress, Orange, Palmarosa or Lemongrass oil**. Mix well to infuse the powder.
- Apply on a damp sponge and use as your surface cleaner, enjoying the aromas as you clean.

Dish Washing-Disinfecting
- For sparkling dishes, add 1 to 2 tablespoons of **Thieves Household Cleaner**, along with **2 to 3 drops of Lemon, Lime, Orange or Melrose** oil. It will create a great smelling kitchen by diffusing the oils this way. Beneficial to inhale while washing.
- **Disinfect** your dishes: Soak your dishes for a few minutes with the above oils – this will also help in ridding bacteria that thrives on dishes.
- Or Make dishwasher detergent by adding 3 to 4 drops of **Lemon, Citrus Fresh, Lime, Bergamot, Melrose or Orange oil** to washing soda. Will also disinfect.

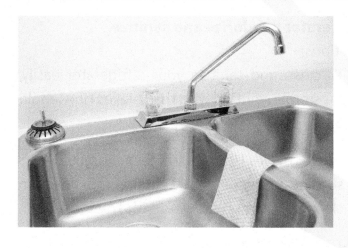

Remember: Disinfect the Sink

Multiple studies have shown that kitchen sinks, including the faucet handles, have extremely **high bacteria counts**. To reduce your risk, here is your 'scents- able' solution.

Thoroughly wash the sink— and faucet handles by spraying your essential oils of Oregano, Lemongrass, Palmarosa, Lemon, Xiang Mao or Thyme. Then use hot, soapy Thieves cleaner water made by diluting your Thieves household cleaner. Rinse well and air dry.

Oven Cleaner

- Clean your oven soon after a spill with moistened baking soda with essential oils.

Directions:

Add 3 drops of **Lavender, Lemon, Lemongrass or Tangerine** oil to your baking soda. Let stand until softened and wipe clean. Repeat if needed.

Then add a few drops of Lemon oil and let stand for a few more minutes - wipe clean.

Rubbish Bins

- Clean, deodorize and disinfect with hot water and disinfecting essential oils.

Directions:

1. Add 4 cups of hot water into your rubbish bin with 3 to 4 drops of any of these oils: Eucalyptus, Melaleuca, Melrose, Lemongrass or Oregano. Let stand to disinfect. Rinse and air dry.
2. Deodorize by adding one drop of the above oils into the bin every now and then (at least 2-3 x weekly).
3. Spray your bin 3x weekly with your spray bottle of oregano, lemongrass or melaleuca oil.

Refrigerator deodorize and sanitize
Directions:

•   To clean and sanitize your refrigerator easily, use this simple solution with the Thieves Household Cleaner.

•   Spray Thieves Household Cleaner on the doors and shelves and wipe with a damp cloth. You can also clean shelves and drawers with Thieves wipes.

•   To fight odors and deodorize then add 3-4 drops of Grapefruit, Orange, Bergamot, Lemongrass or Lemon oil to a wet cloth, then wipe the shelves. The oils help to prevent odours from penetrating other foods as well.

• Add 5 to 10 drops of Lemon, Orange, Tangerine, Bergamot or Palmarosa into a half cup of baking soda. Leave in the refrigerator as a natural absorbent for foul smells.

Some secrets to know about your refrigerator!
Dark, damp environments are the perfect breeding grounds for germs and refrigerators offer such environments such as:

• Refrigerator water dispensers
• Refrigerator vegetable compartments
• Refrigerator ice dispensers
• Refrigerator meat compartments
• Refrigerator insulating seals

It's easy to handle with essential oils.

Spray the vegetable and meat compartments, insulating seals and dispensers several times throughout the week and wipe clean.

Thieves wipes comes in handy in keeping this task simple and hygienic. Simply wipe the areas of concern.

Other areas that harbour germs in the kitchen are: Rubber spatulas, Blenders, Knife blocks, Rubber seals of food storage containers, Can openers.

Directions to sanitize other areas:

For these items: Soak spatulas, and can openers in hot water with 2 drops of each essential oil- Melrose, Lemongrass, Lemon.

For Blenders and knife blocks: Wipe with a damp cloth saturated with essential oils as in wiping the refrigerator.

The CDC listed the top 10 most contaminated areas found in a kitchen starting with the highest germ count on the list ... your refrigerator is number one on the list!

- Refrigerator water dispensers
- Rubber spatulas
- Blenders
- Refrigerator vegetable compartments
- Refrigerator ice dispensers
- Refrigerator meat compartments
- Knife blocks
- Rubber seals of food storage containers
- Can openers
- Refrigerator insulating seals

Water Purification

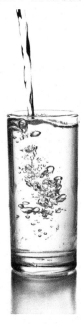

- To a gallon of water, add 4 to 6 drops of Peppermint, Oregano, or Mountain Savoury, Thieves, Orange, Lemon, Clove or Cinnamon oil. Anyone of these oils will help purify your water as well as make your water taste great! These natural flavorings will provide many benefits to your body. Of course, toxic and or polluted water needs to be filtered first and there are many notable companies today that offer powerful and even portable water filters. (see index)

- Distilled water washes out of your system. With the help of essential oils in distilled water, the body can excrete petroleum residues, metals and inorganic minerals, and other toxins.

- One drop per glass is generally enough. Put the oil in first and than add the water. Since oil does not mix with water, putting the oil in first will help disperse it throughout the water.

Some Tips on Greening your drinking water at Restaurants

Any of the above mentioned essential oils can help to purify a glass of drinking water in a restaurant- be it from a water bottle or from the faucet. By adding a drop or two of peppermint essential oil, one can even remove nitrates from your drinking water.

Add Lemon, Lime or Oregano oil (for very unsure water contamination).

Add DiGize blend to aid in digestion and in helping to remove heavy metals, pesticides, bacteria &/or parasites.

How to preserve water for Long-term Storage

Young Living's standard Lemon essential oil is a great way for keeping water clean and fresh for long term water storage and at the same time, helps the water to taste great. (Thieves can be used as well as Oregano).

It's simple enough to do – add 5-7 drops or more of lemon essential oil into 5 gallons of water. This helps to ward off bacterial growth as well as prevent mildew from growing.

Wash – disinfect your knives

A startling 2014 report was recently posted by the Centres for Disease Control and Prevention. After scouring more than 10 years' worth of data about foodborne illness outbreaks, researchers said that norovirus—the awful stomach bug that causes vomiting and diarrhea and that led to so many hospitalizations during the winter of 2014 —is responsible for more illness, by far, than any other pathogen (disease-causing agent).

And about half of foodborne illnesses originate from foods that we usually (and rightly) think of as healthful—specifically, from fresh fruits and vegetables as previously mentioned in Chapter 1.

Before handling raw fruits and vegetables...Do this!

Wash your hands in warm, soapy water (Thieves cleaner or rub 2-3 drops of lemon oil) for at least 20 seconds.

Clean knives and other kitchenware (cutting board, colander, scrub brush) prior to each use by running them through the dishwasher or washing them well with Thieves soap and water. Scrub brushes and dishcloths can be soaked in a solution of a bowl of water with added 3-5 drops of Lemon, Orange, Oregano, Lemongrass, or Citrus Fresh essential oils.

How to wash produce...

Remove and discard outer green leaves from lettuce, cabbage and cauliflower before washing. Wash produce just prior to using or cooking (washing it before storing promotes spoilage).

Use the cleaning tips listed below for soaking produce, as outlined by home expert Cheryl Luptowski (1) with my additions of including essential oils in the wash.

1. Thoroughly wash all produce, including produce that has been organically grown, purchased from a farmers' market or even picked from your own garden. Also wash fruits and vegetables with tough rinds or skins that you won't end up eating—you don't want pathogens to transfer from the food's surface to the knife and then into the flesh upon slicing.

2. Don't plop fruits and veggies in the sink while you wash them—sinks harbour lots of germs. Instead, hold produce in your hands or place the produce in a colander to wash- and spritz the essential oils of Lemon, Orange, Bergamot, Purification, Thieves, Lime, or Citrus Fresh on the fruit and veggies beforehand as well as afterward.

3. Wash produce under running water—it doesn't matter if it is hot or cold. How long you should wash depends (for instance, on the size of what you're washing), but the point is to be thorough. Rub briskly with your hands to help remove dirt and surface microorganisms...for produce that has a firm skin or a rind, such as squash or melon, scrub with a clean brush (that has been soaked in lemon oil or Thieves oil) under running water.

Spritz the produce afterwards.

More in Soaking Fruits and Vegetables

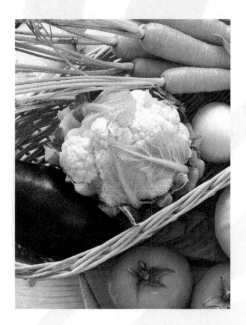

Did you know that by using citrus essential oils – you can clean your fruits and vegetables quite effectively?

Simply fill a bowl with water and add 3-4 drops of Lemon, Lime, Orange, Bergamot, DiGize or Citrus Fresh essential oil to the water. Then add your fruit and vegetables to sit for 10 minutes.

Why? The citrus oils help to dissolve the pesticide residues etc. on the produce. It will also help to lengthen the shelf life as well.

Another alternative:

Use apple cider vinegar to wash your fruits and vegetables - add 3 drops **lemon, Citrus Fresh or Thieves oil** to a bowl of water along with 1 tablespoon of apple cider vinegar.

Another recipe for produce cleansing:

Add a few drops of essential oils of *Lemon, Thieves, Lime, Orange, DiGize, Bergamot or Purification* to a bowl filled with cold water- with 2 tablespoons of **Thieves household cleaner**.

Soak your fruits and vegetables for a few minutes as this will help to wash off parasites; help fruits & vegetables store longer and breakdown the wax.

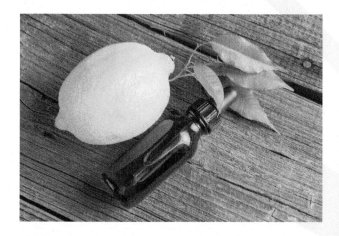

Did you know it takes 3,000 lemons to produce 1 kilo of oil!

Lemon oil is Rich in limonene, which has been extensively studied in over 50 clinical studies for its ability to combat tumor growth.

University researchers of Japan found that diffusing certain aromas in an office environment dramatically improved mental accuracy and concentration. Diffused <u>lemon</u> *resulted in 54% fewer errors, jasmine resulted in 33% fewer errors, and lavender resulted in 20 percent fewer errors. When aromas were diffused during test taking, scores increased by as much as 50%.*

Interesting Properties

- **Prevents toxic chemical build –ups thus supporting a healthy system**

- **Can be used as an antiseptic – a substance which inhibits the growth and development of microorganisms on countertops, sinks, surfaces.**

The Many Benefits of Lemon Essential oil

Can help to support many health conditions and air purification.

Young Living purity standard:

- **air disinfectant**
- **helpful to breathe easier**
- **supports brain focus**
- **helpful for concentration**
- **maintains a healthy positive feeling**
- **immune system booster**
- **supports healthy skin**
- **maintains smooth skin**
- **supports the digestive system**
- **helps as a gum-grease remover on upholstery, furniture, clothing**
- **supports and maintains a healthy urinary system**
- **supports a healthy liver-gallbladder system**
- **calming and relaxing, helps with stress**
- **supports the nervous system**
- **maintains healthy, smooth legs**
- **purifying water and more household uses......**

37

- **Maintains a healthy circulatory system**

- **Supports a healthy immune system**

- **Helps to maintain a healthy brain**

- **Citrus scent is an instant pick-me-up,**

- **Relaxing, refreshing and stimulating**

Stainless Steel Cleaner

- Remove smudges/marks from stainless steel appliances with 3 drops of **Lemon or Purification** oil, added to one tablespoon of olive oil. Mix well. Dip a rag into the oil mixture and rub the surface to rid smudges. Apply vinegar onto another rag – wipe and let dry.

- Did you know that the superbug MRSA can survive on stainless steel for days?

- Wipe your stainless steel with **Melaleuca, Lemon, Oregano, Thyme or Lemongrass oil** at least once or twice a week. Dip your rag into a mixture of several drops of oil in a bowl of water, and wipe your appliance Or simply spray your oil onto the appliance and wipe clean.

- Please note: A July 2012 study conducted at Mississippi State University screened nine essential oils and constituents for their **ability to eliminate biofilms of Listeria monocytogenes on polystyrene and stainless steel surfaces. The highest antimicrobial activity was found with <u>thyme oil, oregano oil and carvacrol. (2)</u>**

FOOD PREPARATION REAL GREEN TIPS TO PREVENT FOOD POISONING!

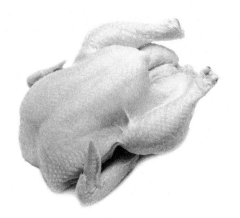

Don't wash that bird-!

Well that is the latest from the Centre of Disease Control!

So what can you do?

I say - **Spritz that bird instead!**

You can use these same essential oils to keep your food safe, healthy and flavorful! Have these oils in your spritzer bottles on hand: **Oregano, Thyme, Orange, Lemon, Bergamot, Lemongrass, Rosemary, Thieves and/or Lime.**

Researchers point out that bacteria and chickens are a dangerous combination. (3) As presented earlier in Chapter 1, foodborne illnesses harbour in kitchens. I also outlined some of the essential oil research that showed their natural anti-bacterial properties.

Two major food pathogens, *Salmonella enteritidis* and *Campylobacter jejuni* can be transmitted to humans through poultry products. A February 2013 study by Venkitanarayanan K, et al., reported that "Chickens are the reservoir hosts of these pathogens, with their intestinal colonization being the most significant factor causing contamination of meat and eggs." (4)

The CDC points out that most people wouldn't think of preparing a chicken or turkey without rinsing the bird first. Unfortunately, it has been found that rinsing does not wash away *Salmonella* or other disease-causing microbes. Instead rinsing poultry is considered by the CDC the worst thing you can do: why? Because it isn't very effective at removing bacteria and it **sprays potentially contaminated water droplets around your kitchen.**

These harmful organisms can survive for days or even weeks on faucets, countertops, the refrigerator handle, etc. They cause cross-contamination when other foods (or your fingers) touch the invisible hot spots. So here is what you can do using the Vibrational

Cleaning methods of kitchen 'scents' quite easily:

Remember that the research on food safety and preservation found a number of oils to be very beneficial and protective.

Create your spray bottles of **oregano, lemon, orange, bergamot, citrus fresh, lemongrass, or thyme oil** to have on your counter top as previously outlined in Chapter 1, by simply adding 10-15 drops of your choice of essential oil into a 8oz spray bottle of water.

a) Spray the bird well with **oregano oil** first and wait for 10 minutes.

b) Then spray with **lemon oil** and wait another 10 minutes- and make sure that the bird is quite saturated with the oil mixture.

c) Now you can rinse your bird and spray again with **Lemon, Thyme, Bergamot, Marjoram or oregano oils**. The benefits are wonderful as the oil spray is not only a food preservative/ protectant but it is also a **food flavouring**. I personally spritz two or three oils afterwards anytime I prepare organic chicken or fish and do the same for all my greens and salads.

c) Spritz the countertop, sink and cutting board as well afterwards then rinse with Thieves cleaner.

Cooking Tip:

Always **cook poultry (whether in your kitchen or on the grill) to an internal temperature of 165°F.** The High temperature—not the rinsing—will ensure that the bird is safe to eat.

Wash your hands *after* handling poultry but better still spray your hands with oregano or lemon oil then wash. Most people remember to wash their hands before handling foods, but it's actually more important to do so *afterwards* as well to prevent the spread of bacteria.

The Cutting Board

The cutting board has been found to be one of the most contaminated surfaces in your kitchen, particularly if you use the same one for all of your food preparations.

The bacteria from poultry and other meats are easily transferred to other foods. Wiping a cutting board with a sponge isn't an effective way to remove microbes.

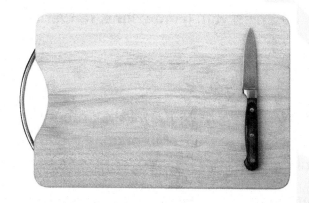

Make sure that your cutting board is washed under running water with Thieves cleaner and then sprayed with **oregano oil, lemongrass, bergamot or citrus Fresh** oil.

Plastic or wood cutting boards Plastic cutting boards are considered less porous and easier to clean. Wood cutting boards have natural bacteria-inhibiting properties in them but also tend to harbour the bacteria in the grains of the wood. Either one is acceptable—but just keep it clean by using hot, **Thieves** cleaner soapy water, or sanitizing it in the dishwasher and spraying the essential oils as mentioned above, let them soak in and air-dry.

To minimize foodborne risks: Every home would be wise to have two cutting boards—one that's used only for poultry/other meats and one that's used only for produce.

Common oversight: Many do not think to wash a knife that was used to cut poultry before cutting other foods. Wash it with hot, Thieves soapy water and then spritz it with **oregano or thyme oil.**

Other helpful Food preparation Tips:

- Add 1 or 2 drops to your recipes towards the end of cooking or your food preparations. This will help to keep the flavor strong. Add as per your favourite taste and recipe: Lemon, Lime, Lavender, Bergamot, Rosemary, Marjoram, Oregano, Peppermint, and Orange or Tangerine oil.

For example:

- Season salad dressings with lemon, oregano, rosemary, or peppermint essential oils

- Infuse your bottle of extra virgin olive oil- by simply adding a few sprigs of fresh herbs of basil , rosemary or oregano and a few drops of Young Living's essential oils: **basil, black pepper, dill, fennel, clove, lemongrass, rosemary, oregano, or thyme**

41

- Season baked goods (frostings, puddings, fruit pies) with **lemon, lime, tangerine, peppermint and/or lavender**

- Create your own **lavender sea salt**-

- Combine a few sprigs of fresh lavender flowers in a bowl if available, otherwise combine 2 drops of lavender oil into 2 cups of Celtic sea salt – Mix or grind together. Delicious on salads, vegetables and/or poultry.

- Marinade your food, your vegetables, fruit, or any meat/fish with added drops of oils: e.g. combine 1- 2 tbsp olive oil, fresh squeezed lemon juice, Bragg's amino or coconut amino mixture with 1 drop oregano or thyme or rosemary essential oil, add chopped fresh herbs to your liking

- Add to hot water for your favorite herbal tea: 1-2 drops of peppermint, spearmint, lemon, or lavender

- Flavour honey or agave with your choice of essential oil including raw cacao. Delicious!

Triple - purpose food spray

As discussed earlier, **oregano and thyme** oil can 1.disinfect your cutting board or countertop, 2.preserve your food and 3. add flavor.

- Simply fill a spray bottle half full with filtered water; add ***20 drops of oregano, thyme, marjoram and/or cinnamon oil;*** shake and spritz where needed.

Remember, since these oils are GRAS approved as food enhancers and Young Living oils are chemical–free & edible, they can be used on your ***food for flavouring, as your disinfecting cleanser agent as well as your food preservative! So Bon Appétit!***

CHAPTER 3

Bathroom scents

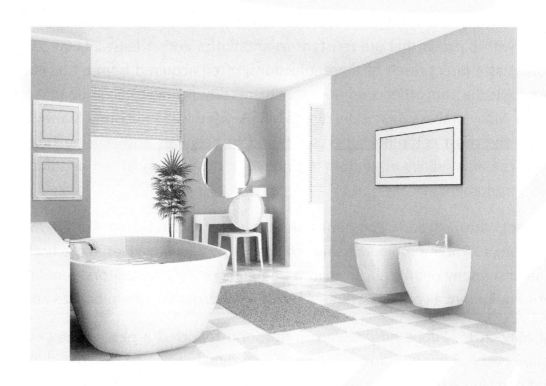

A perfumed bath and a scented massage every day is the way to good health"

Hippocrates 400 BC

GREEN YOUR BATHROOM CABINET TOO!

SUPERBUGS-A GROWING GLOBAL PROBLEM
KEEP YOUR BATHROOM FREE OF BACTERIA & MOLD!

In the battle against harmful bacteria and germs, the overuse of antibiotics and antibacteriacides (household and industrial cleansers) has created a growing global problem with antibiotic resistant bacteria that we have no solution for. Those individuals who contract the disease are often left without any treatment options. The more antibiotics that are used, the more the bacteria become resistant to them. The regular misuse and overuse of antibiotics and vaccines have been a major contributing factor to the creation of "superbugs" including broad spectrum antibacteriacidal agents such as Triclosan (more on triclosan in 'Vibrational Cleaning' book).

Each year as reported by the CDC in the United States, at least 2 million people become infected with bacteria that are resistant to antibiotics and at least 23,000 people die each year as a direct result of these infections, often acquired from a hospital. Many more people die from other conditions that were complicated by an antibiotic-resistant infection. Many of these deaths are due to MRSA - Methicillin-Resistant Staphylococcus Aureus - the most common 'superbug' found in hospitals and nursing homes. The bacteria can also survive away from the body - in dust, in unwashed bedding and on medical equipment. (1)

For patients, the most dangerous time is during surgery when there are open wounds for the bacteria to enter the bloodstream. Ironically, the very advances in medical science that keep so many people alive can also be a danger. Drips, monitors, ventilators and dialysis equipment all provide avenues for bacteria to get into the bloodstream. (2)

As of May, 2014, Public hospitals in Hong Kong reported a new case of superbug infection every 18 minutes during last year, according to Hospital Authority figures and Hong Kong University microbiologist Dr Ho Pak-leung. The statistics show an overall 15 per cent increase in three major types of superbug infection from 2011. (3)

Anti-biotic resistant bacteria have become a concern worldwide. Once again we have proven effectiveness in essential oils research outlining their Super-Powerful benefits.

FABULOUS DISCOVERY- SUPERBUG PROTECTION

Essential oils work better for Superbugs than do drugs!

In March 2013, the Centers for Disease Control and Prevention (CDC) sounded the alarm on the deadly family of "nightmare" untreatable superbugs as they spread throughout U.S. hospitals.

This is often the alternative that hospitals are now facing re the superbug endemic:

"I've had to ask patients, 'Do you want a toxic antibiotic and end up on dialysis, or would you prefer to have a limb amputated?'" Dr. Fishman said. There is little chance that an effective drug to kill CRE bacteria will be produced in the coming years. Manufacturers have no new antibiotics in development that show promise, according to federal officials and industry experts, and there's little financial incentive because the bacteria adapt quickly to resist new drugs.!! This is the state of medicine today- it's in crisis! (4)

*Critical News to our rescue: In a recent study, natural essential oils—including **tea tree oil** were found to be more effective at killing super bugs than standard disinfectants.*

Mother Nature's plant wisdom offers us the answers- Researchers from Australia's Royal Brisbane and Women's Hospital tested a number of plant extracts, including **tea tree, lemongrass and eucalyptus,** against several of the most deadly antibiotic-resistant superbugs. These included:

- **Klebsiella pneumoniae**

- **MRSA (methicillin-resistant Staphylococcus aureus)**

- **VRE (vancomycin-resistant Enterococcus)**

- **Multi-drug resistant Pseudomonas aeruginosa**

- **ESBL-producing Escherichia coli**

They also tested these strains against two common antiseptics often used in hospitals—chlorhexidine and ethanol, commonly termed rubbing alcohol. They then looked at the "zone of inhibition," which is the distance the substance will repel the bug, preventing infection. A larger zone meant the substance was a stronger antiseptic.

Results showed:

- Rubbing alcohol had "notably lower or no efficacy in regard to growth inhibition of strains."

- **Lemongrass, eucalyptus, and tea tree oils** had large zones of inhibition—significantly greater than the rubbing alcohol.

- **Lemongrass oil** significantly inhibited gram-positive bacteria, while **tea tree oil** significantly inhibited gram-negative bacteria. Klebsiella pneumoniae, enterococcus and pseudomonas aeruginosa which are all gram-negative bacteria while **staphylococcus aureus is a gram-positive bacterium. (4) (5)**

The first essential oil study showing efficacy against MRSA was published in March 1995. Australian researchers turned to their "home-town favorite" Melaleuca alternifolia. The research showed all 66 isolates of Staphylococcus aureus were susceptible to the essential oil in disc diffusion and modified broth micro dilution methods. Sixty-four of the isolates tested were methicillin-resistant S. aureus (MRSA), and 33 were mupirocin-resistant.

- Melaleuca, Lavender, peppermint and thyme essential oils showed the strongest killing power against MRSA and VRE antibiotic-resistant bacteria, according to studies at the Western Infirmary, Glasgow, UK.

- A 2012 study - also added another essential oil to the list: **Lemongrass which was found to be 100% effective.**

Another group of researchers stated that essential oil vapors are able to reduce environmental bacterial contamination. They tested a vaporized blend of citrus essential oils *(orange and bergamot)* to remove Enterococcus sp. and S. aureus from stainless steel surfaces and saw its effect on the formation of bacterial biofilms. Both oils were impressive in that "Staphyloccocal biofilms were reduced both during and after formation, whereas enterococcal biofilms were significantly reduced only after formation…. The researchers concluded that Citrus vapour has potential for application in the clinical environment. (6)

Pub Med (website of the National Library of Medicine) shows nearly **200 scientific essential** oil studies that have investigated the following well-known oils against drug-resistant (MRSA) pathogens:

- A blend of *Melaleuca alternifolia,* peppermint, eucalyptus and cajuput;

- an orange/bergamot vapor;

- thyme, clove, cinnamon bark, coriander, oregano, lavender, grapefruit, sage, lemon, lemongrass,

- a geranium-lemongrass blend,

- a geranium-tea tree blend,

- lemon myrtle, spearmint

- Japanese mint, helichrysum, rosemary, ginger, hyssop, sandalwood and a number of exotic essential oils from places as diverse as Turkey and Yemen.

Science Daily reported that Essential oils could be a cheap and effective alternative to antibiotics and they can potentially be used to combat drug-resistant hospital superbugs, according to research presented at the Society for General Microbiology's spring meeting in 2010 Edinburgh.

The lead researchers Professor Yiannis Samaras and Dr Effimia Eriotou, from the Technological Educational Institute of Ionian Islands, in Greece, tested the antimicrobial activity of eight plant essential oils with amazing results. According to their findings, **Thyme essential oil was the most effective and was able to almost completely eliminate bacteria within 60 minutes.**

They also discovered that the essential oils of **_thyme and cinnamon_ were particularly efficient antibacterial agents against a range of Staphylococcus species.** These bacteria strains are common inhabitants of the skin and some may cause infection in immuno-compromised individuals. Drug-resistant strains, such as methicillin-resistant *Staphylococcus aureus* (MRSA) are extremely difficult to treat. *"Not only are essential oils a cheap and effective treatment option for antibiotic-resistant strains, but decreased use of antibiotics will help minimise the risk of new strains of antibiotic resistant micro-organisms emerging," said Professor Samaras.*

The Greek researchers believe that essential oils could have diverse medical and industrial

47

applications. "The oils -- or their active ingredients -- could be easily incorporated into antimicrobial creams or gels for external application. In the food industry the impregnation of food packaging with essential oils has already been successfully trialled. They could also be included in food stuffs to replace synthetic chemicals that act as preservatives," they said. (Published in Science Daily, April 4, 2010) (7)

I find it alarming that the world at large doesn't seem to be well informed of the efficacy of essential oils against the superbugs that now lurk not only in hospitals but throughout our communities as well. *Locker rooms, gyms and wrestling mats have sent professional athletes* as well as high school and college sports' stars to the emergency room. "Community-acquired" infections are becoming as prevalent as the hospital-acquired infections. So having this guidebook in your hands is your guide to greater health, safety and peace of mind and one that you can now inform others about, to help safeguard their lives.

General Cleaning Tip reminders:

- **Get rid of the triclosan: It's in a number of antibacterial soaps and cleaners, yet it's been linked to the increase in superbugs. It also contaminates the environment, polluting rivers and lakes.**

- **Use the homemade cleaners suggested in this guidebook:**

- **Make your own hand sanitizer: Add one or more of these oils to water in a sprayer or other small bottle, shake, and apply to clean hands between washings.**

General bathroom cleaner with 100% Essential oil power

- Use any of the following oils as a room spray or surface cleaner: **Oregano, Thyme, Orange, Bergamot, Lemon, Lemongrass, Palmarosa, Eucalyptus, Melaleuca (Tea Tree) or Lavender or the blend called Melrose™.**

Directions:

- Apply 2 to 3 drops directly onto a wet wash cloth, or use 8 – 10 drops in 2 litres of washing water. Dip your wash cloth and wipe surfaces clean.

- Apply 3-4 drops of **Oregano** oil on a damp wash cloth to disinfect countertops and sinks. Better still, use the oil of **Lemongrass** (3 drops) on damp cloth first for the gram positive staphylococcus bacteria then follow with a few sprays of **Melaleuca** oil for the gram negative bacteria.!

- Mix 10 drops of **Melaleuca** oil in an 8 ounce spray bottle of water

All-purpose cleaning-disinfecting spray

- For tiles, countertops, floors, tubs. To one gallon of hot water, add ½ cup of white vinegar, 1 tablespoon of Borax, and 15 drops of **Lemongrass, Oregano, Thyme, Lemon, Orange, Thieves (contains cinnamon) or Palmarosa oil, or Xiang Mao**.

Green Disinfectant

- Mix 50 to 100 drops of **Eucalyptus oil** with a litre of water. Shake and use in a spray bottle. Eucalyptus oil is a good disinfectant and deodorizer. It gets rid of some stains like ink and grease, kills and repels some insects. ***It'll even attack rust.***

- Disinfect wash cloths by soaking them in a bowl of boiling water with 2-3 drops of **Eucalyptus, Lavender, Purification, Melaleuca, Thyme, Oregano, or Citrus Fresh** oil before washing.

- Disinfectant blend: To a small bowl of water, add 2 drops of **Lavender oil, 4 drops of Thyme oil, 1 drop of Eucalyptus oil and 1 drop of Oregano oil.**

- **Lemon, Spruce, or Fir oil** can also be used for disinfecting bathrooms and kitchens.

- Soak toothbrushes in solution of **Oregano oil, Thieves oil, Melrose oil or Melaleuca** oil in salted water to combat microbes. Add a couple of drops to your toothbrush with Thieves toothpaste.

49

Toilets

- Use **Oregano oil** for disinfecting toilets. Add a drop every day.

- Use 2 to 3 drops of **Lemon, Citrus Fresh and Palmarosa or Eucalyptus oil** for cleaning. Scrub toilet and let stand a few minutes.

- Can also use **Melaleuca, Melrose, Lemongrass or Purification** oil for toilets by applying 2 drops into the toilet bowl, let stand for 5 minutes or longer and then flush: can also apply a few drops on the inside of your toilet paper roll as well.

Toilet Cleaner Formula

- Ingredients:

- 25 drops melaleuca or Melrose blend

- 1 cup water in a spray bottle

- Instructions:

- Add oil and water to spray bottle.

- Shake, then spritz along the toilet's inside rim and bowl

- Let sit for 30 minutes; scrub and rinse

Mold Remediation

- Found mold in your shower stall? Mold is often found in bathrooms and kitchens – but can happen anywhere there is a leak.

- Steps to *remediating Mold are found in Chapter 5.*

- Your Thieves household cleaner and Thieves oil blend will be most useful for this job.

Air fresheners

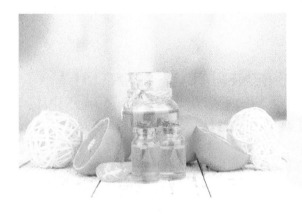

Directions:

•   Use 2 drops of **Lemon, Purification, Rosemary, Melaleuca, Eucalyptus or Grapefruit oil** or **Xiang Mao** on the cardboard inner ring of your toilet paper roll.

•   Create your own natural potpourri with dried flowers by adding oils of your choice throughout your home or office.

• For a deodorizing spray, mix **2 drops Rosemary, 4 drops Lemon, 3 drops Eucalyptus and 4 drops Lavender** in 1 quart of water. Shake well and spray where needed.

Choose healthier, natural ways to fill your 'bathroom' cabinet – make it instead a **'Supportive- Green ' cabinet.**

Please note: The statements below for ***Greening your bathroom cabinet*** have not been evaluated by the FDA. The products listed are not intended to diagnose, treat, cure or prevent any disease. They are merely educational. Seek proper medical help and consult with your health care practitioner of your choice.

MAKE YOUR BATHROOM CABINET A 'SUPPORTIVE GREEN' CABINET

CREATE AN ALL NATURAL WAY TO USE BENEFICIAL ESSENTIAL OILS TO SUPPORT MANY BODILY SYSTEMS, COMPARED TO USING HARMFUL CHEMICALS FOUND IN YOUR TYPICAL BATHROOM PRODUCTS.

EVERYDAY ESSENTIAL OILS FOR A WELLNESS LIFESTYLE

Frankincense	Can use these supportive oils Spiritual Awakener	• Calming properties that can increase spiritual connection and inner strength. • Helps to support healthy skin, • The ancient Egyptians used the oil found in the wild-crafted resin of Boswellia carteri trees in Kenya to promote younger, fresher looking skin.
Lemon	Refreshing Cleanser	• Cold pressed from the fresh fruit peel of lemons grown in Argentina and the United States, lemon oil has refreshing and cooling properties. • Its fresh, citrus scent is an instant pick-me-up. • Supports the nervous, digestive and immune systems

Lavender	Fragrant Supporter	• Steam distilled from the flowering plants grown at the Young Living farms in Simiane-la-Rotonde, France, and Mona, Utah, lavender is the most versatile essential oil. • Use For: • Skin Irritations • Balancing • •Relaxing • •Its refreshing, relaxing scent has balancing properties that also bring a sense of calm. • •Supports restful sleep • Use for promoting younger, fresher looking skin.
Peace & Calming	The Peacemaker tangerine, ylang ylang, blue tansy, orange, patchouli	• The gentle scent of Peace & Calming® encourages deep relaxation and may assist with meditation prior to bedtime. • Promotes and supports peaceful feelings in children and pets.
PanAway	Comfort Restorer wintergreen, clove, helichrysum, peppermint	• PanAway® contains wintergreen and clove essential oils. These oils or their active components are widely used in massage after physical activity. • Supports healthy muscle • Supports healthy joint and cartilage function
Valor	Brave Heart spruce, blue tansy, frankincense	• Valor® is an empowering blend that promotes feelings of strength, courage, confidence and protection. • Valor is also believed to support energy alignment.

53

Thieves	Protector clove, cinnamon bark, rosemary, lemon, eucalyptus (E. radiata)	• The revolutionary Thieves® blend contains powerful essential oils that have many household and personal uses. • Diffuse throughout the home to neutralize unwanted odors, mildew, Mold or apply to the bottoms of the feet. • Supports the immune system and to maintain healthy teeth and gums
Peppermint	Madam Cool	• One of the oldest and most highly regarded herbs, peppermint essential oil has a fresh aroma that is energizing to give you a renewed feeling of vigor. • Supports normal, healthy digestion • Supports and maintains focus & concentration
Purification	Purifier	• The sweet refreshing scent of Purification® instantly deodorizes unpleasant odors in the air. • This blend also contains citronella oil. • Many personal outdoor uses. • Soothes annoying irritations

CHAPTER 4

Laundry Scents

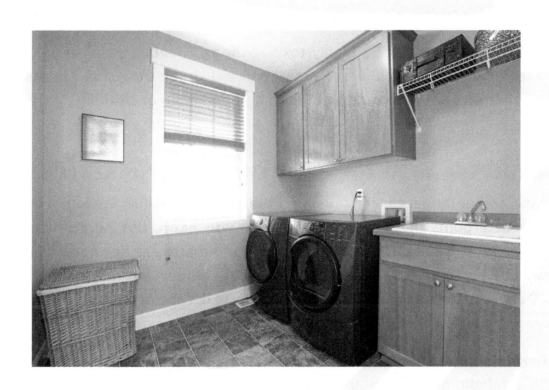

*"Smells are surer than sounds or sights
to make your heart strings crack"*

Rudyard Kipling

TOXIC DETERGENTS - TOXIC CLOTHING

What's lurking on your freshly washed clothes? What's lurking in your laundry room? Much of this information on toxic laundry detergents was detailed in my first book, so here is a quick overview of the toxic detergents that most families use, not ever realizing that the chemicals in laundry detergents leave a residue and a perfumed smell that threatens you and your family's health in a way you may never have imagined!

Unfortunately, **most laundry detergents contain a potentially toxic brew of chemicals that can leave residues behind on your clothing, be absorbed by your skin or be released into the air you breathe.** Dryer sheets for example, coat all your clothes with a layer of toxic chemicals. When you wear those clothes, your body moisture causes those chemicals to come into contact with your skin and be absorbed directly into your bloodstream. It's an easy way to poison your system with cancer-causing chemicals.

The laundry room becomes a highly toxic room as it harbours the same chemical perfumes released by the **laundry detergent** and **dryer sheets. It can also hold bacteria or microbes that could be hidden in soiled linen or clothing.**

REMINDERS OF A FEW TOXIC AND CARCINOGENIC CHEMICALS

The toxic and potential cancer-causing chemicals listed below are found in typical laundry detergents that can not only cause you harm, but raise havoc in the environment as well. Most are cancer-causing and also are hormone disruptors. These harsh chemicals can build up in your clothes and eventually penetrate your skin. Detergent makers are not required by law to list any of these ingredients. For a more detailed list, please refer to Vibrational Cleaning book.

- **Dioxane (1,4-dioxane)** – The majority of top laundry detergent brands contain this synthetic petrochemical, a serious known carcinogen. This is a by-product contaminant of the manufacturing process and is not required to be listed on product labels.

- **Linear alky benzene sulfonates (LAS)** – Synthetic petrochemicals that biodegrade slowly making them an environmental hazard. Benzene may cause cancer in humans and animals.

- **Artificial fragrances** – Linked to various toxic effects on fish and mammals, and can cause allergies, skin and eye irritation to humans.

- **Phosphates** – Used to prevent dirt from settling back into clothes after being washed. Can stimulate growth of marine plants that trigger unbalanced ecosystems.

MORE REMINDERS ABOUT THE DANGERS OF 1,4-DIOXANE

As outlined from my Vibrational Cleaning book:

"**1,4-dioxane is a synthetic petrochemical carcinogen,** created when laundry detergents and other cleaning products are cheaply manufactured using ethoxylation (a short-cut industrial process in which ethylene oxide is added to fatty acid alcohols to give them detergent properties).

In 2010, Green Patriot Working Group and the Organic Consumers Association published the results of a study on 1,4 dioxane levels in laundry detergents. About two thirds of the detergents tested contained 1,4 dioxane. Thirteen of them were popular brands, one of which had levels as high as 55 ppm.

Traditionally, our ancestors used flowers, shrubs or bushes to scent their laundry in order to have fresh, clean-smelling clothes. They would dry their clothes on rosemary or lavender bushes to scent them. Lavender is known for its fresh scent and melaleuca for its disinfecting power.

Now you can once again scent your clothes with Nature's aromatic gifts – No more chemicals!

LAUNDRY ROOM SANITATION

- **Add 2 or 3 drops** of **lemon oil** to water and spray the laundry room, counter tops and sinks as **lemon oil** will help sanitize the entire room.

- Use other oils like **Thieves, Oregano, Thyme, Palmarosa, Lavender or Melrose**

- Wipe the countertops and sinks with the **Thieves** handi-wipes or wash with the Thieves Household cleaner

WASHING YOUR CLOTHES

Add essential oils to your laundry to increase anti-bacterial benefits and to provide greater hygiene.

- **Use Thieves Household Cleaner in your wash water. Simply add 1 – 2 capfuls depending on your wash load.**

- **Recent research has shown that _Eucalyptus oil kills dust mites_. Dust mites live in your bedding, feeding from the dead skin cells you constantly shed.** To kill dust mites, add 25 drops of Eucalyptus oil to each wash load.

- As a softening agent, add a dampened wash cloth loaded with 10 drops of **Lavender, Lemon, or Melaleuca oil.**

- Add a couple of drops of **Lemon, Lavender, Rosemary, Purification, Lemongrass, Citrus Fresh or Bergamot** oil to the final rinse water.

- Add 2 to 3 drops of **Lavender, Joy, Palmarosa, or Bergamot** oil directly to the clothes in your dryer, or on a small cloth.

- Soak your dishcloth or other laundry items overnight in a bowl of water with **a few drops** of lemon oil to help to sanitize them.

- Use a drop or two of lemon essential oil on stains. Let stand, and rub off with a clean cloth or throw into laundry cycle. **Lemon oil can also** help remove gum, oil, grease spots or crayon marks.

SPECIFIC CLOTHES SANITATION

Any linen, bedclothes and clothes that have been soiled (excrement) from any sick family member with bacterial enteritis (including secondary infection) should be washed with sanitizing essential oils:

Directions:

Add 2 caps of Thieves detergent undiluted along with 25 drops of Thieves oil or Oregano Oil in hot water of 80 degrees centigrade for 10 minutes.

Then continue to wash and rinse.

Butter or Oil Stain Remover

- 1 tablespoon baking soda

- 2 drops Lemon, Lime or Grapefruit Oil

- Water

Directions:

- Make a paste and apply to stain.

- Allow to dry then wash.

Stain Remover

- Ingredients:

- 1 tablespoon cornstarch

- 2- 3 Drops of Eucalyptus Essential Oil

- 1 teaspoon glycerin

Directions:

1. Make into a paste

2. Spread on stain and allow garment to dry.

3. Reapply until stain is gone then launder.

Or Can also soak the garment in Thieves cleaner with Eucalyptus Oil

Directions:

Add a capful or two of Thieves cleaner into your laundry tub with 10 drops of Eucalyptus Essential oil. Soak for at least 30 minutes or longer.

Clothes Dryer:

Add essential oils for freshening and deodorizing your clothing

Directions:

- Add **Thieves wipes** to your dryer. simply throw in one or two sheets in the dryer

- Instead of using toxic and irritating softening sheets in the dryer, toss in a dampened washcloth with 10 **drops of lavender, lemon, melaleuca, bergamot**, or other oils that you'd like to add. While the oils will not reduce static cling, they will impart a lovely, clean, refreshing fragrance to your clothes.

- To help create natural clothing pest repellent- then add drops of **lavender, Purification, Eucalyptus, or Lemongrass t**o your dryer. It's a great way to have your clothes smell clean and fresh that act as an insect deterrent as well.

Simple no-fuss **static cling solution**

- simply roll aluminum foil into a ball and throw it in your dryer.

ALTERNATIVES TO MOTH BALLS FOR PROTECTING YOUR CLOTHING

First of all- the toxic dangers of moth balls (consisting of naphthalene) are much more known today but many still opt to use this poisonous chemical. Naphthalene is an incredibly dangerous chemical. According to the Material Safety Data Sheet (MSDS) required by the Occupational Safety and Health Association (OHSA) to list dangerous chemicals, it outlines naphthalene's dangers.

MSDS warns that naphthalene is harmful if swallowed or inhaled; it causes irritation to skin, eyes and respiratory tract, and may affect liver, kidney, blood and central nervous system. Furthermore, MSDS states that inhalation of dust or vapors can cause headache, nausea, vomiting, extensive sweating and disorientation. It further points out that the predominant reaction is delayed intravascular haemolysis (the dissolution of red blood cells) with symptoms of anemia, fever, jaundice and kidney or liver damage. So using moth balls is a hefty price to pay with your health in order to protect your clothing.

ESSENTIAL OILS INSTEAD AS MOTH REPELLENT

Easy to make your own natural mothballs

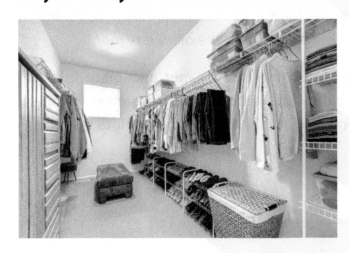

Directions:

• Simply soak cotton wool balls in a repelling essential oil: such as **Cedarwood, lavender, rosemary, lemongrass, clove or eucalyptus**. When the balls feel dry, scatter them in amongst your clothes drawers.

• Refresh the balls every couple of months.

• Scatter dried herbs (e.g. cedar chips, rosemary, lavender, cloves) with drops of the essential oils placed under porous paper drawer liners

MAKE YOUR OWN MOTH REPELLING SACHETS

Add cedar chips or dried lavender flowers to cotton muslin and wrap to create a ball or use a cotton bag. Apply several drops of the repelling essential oils of **Cedarwood, rosemary, lavender or clove**. Can also use cotton balls soaked in the oils and place where needed.

CLOSETS – WARDROBE
DEODORIZE YOUR CLOSETS

Make your linens smell fresh by adding oils to the cupboard liner or strips of blotting paper.

Directions:

• Add several drops of **Lavender, Chamomile, Marjoram, Rosemary or Palmarosa** to a strip of blotting paper- then hang in closet

• For fresh and moth-free clothes, spray a few drops of **Lavender** or **Eucalyptus** into the closets and drawers.

Moth repellant Directions:

- Make a sachet by placing several drops of **Citronella, Lavender, Lemongrass or Rosemary** oil on a cotton ball. Wrap and tie it into a small handkerchief. Hang in storage areas in your closet, remember to refresh with the oils every month.

- Deodorize smelly shoes: Add oil to strips of blotting paper and place in shoes overnight. Use 2 to 3 drops of **Eucalyptus, Lemongrass, Bergamot, Cypress, Lavender and /or Purification.** The oils can also be applied directly into the shoes.

CHAPTER 5

General Cleaning Scents and Steps to Cleaning Mold

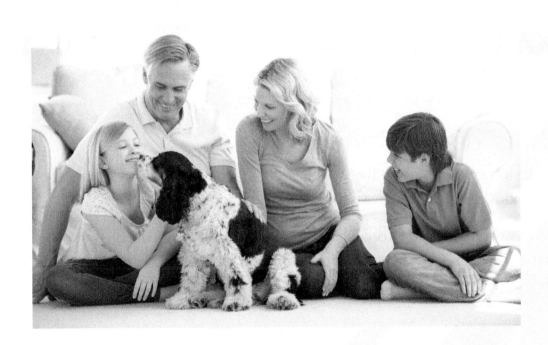

"The garden of the heart is moist and fresh with jasmines, rose and cypress trees."

Rumi

GENERAL HOUSEHOLD CLEANING TIPS

Disinfect anywhere in the home/office with Thieves Wipes

- **Thieves Wipes** are ideal for use on door handles, toilet seats and any surface that needs cleaning to protect from dust, mold, and undesirable microorganisms. Keep a pack handy in your bathroom, laundry room, kitchen, car, office, or anywhere else you want to keep your environment clean without toxic chemicals.

- Thieves essential oil blend (contains clove, cinnamon, eucalyptus, lemon and rosemary oils) has been university tested for its effects against unwanted microorganisms and found to be highly effective in supporting the immune system and good health. (More details found in Chapter 3 Vibrational Cleaning book)

FURNITURE POLISH

- In a spray bottle, combine ½ cup of vegetable oil with 2 tablespoons of white or cleaning vinegar and 10 to 15 drops of **Spruce, Cedarwood, Cypress, Fir, Lemon, Vetiver or Lavender** oil. Shake, spray and polish with a rag. Test on the wood beforehand.

MIRRORS, GLASS, WINDOWS

- Make a cleaning spray with equal parts vinegar and water, and **10 drops of Lemon, Lime or Grapefruit oil**. Use a paper or microfiber towel.

- After washing, add one drop of **Lemon, Lime or Grapefruit** oil to a newspaper or paper towel and rub over windows to remove streaky marks. Or use the formula below

GLASS CLEANER

Ingredients:

- 1 tablespoon white vinegar

- 1 quart of water

- 10 drops lemon essential oil

- Spray bottle

Combine in a spray bottle. Shake before each use.

HARDWOOD FLOORS AND CARPETS

- Hardwood floors: Add ¼ cup white vinegar to a bucket of water. Add 5 to 10 drops of **Lemon, Cedarwood or Fir** oil. OR ***Brain Power, Inspiration or Into The Future***

- Carpet freshener: Add 16 to 20 drops of **Lemon, Citrus Fresh, Lavender or Bergamot oil** to a cup of baking soda. Mix well and cover overnight. Then sprinkle it over your carpet, wait 10 minutes and vacuum.

SPECIAL DEODORIZING SPRAY

This spray deodorizes and cleans the air instead of masking the odors—a real odor eater!

Ingredients:

- 2 drops rosemary essential oil

- 4 drops lemon essential oil

- 2 drops eucalyptus (E. globulus) essential oil

- 4 drops lavender essential oil

- 1 quart distilled water or purified water

Fill a 1 quart spray bottle with water, add the essential oils and mix by shaking the bottle. Use to clean the air or even on countertops, sinks, tiles or cupboards.

HOT TUBS AND SAUNAS:

- Use 3 drops per person of **lavender, cinnamon, clove, eucalyptus, geranium, thyme, lemon,** or **grapefruit** essential oil to disinfect and freshen the water. Can add **Brain Power, Sacred Frankincense or Inspiration**

- For saunas, add several drops of **rosemary, thyme, pine, or lavender** oil to a spray bottle with water, and spray surfaces. This water can also be used to splash onto hot sauna stones.

AIR FRESHENING

You can use any essential oil as an air freshener to gain its therapeutic benefits. See the Index of Essential Oils to learn more, or use one of my favorites:

- **Lavender**: improves sleep quality and calms the nervous system

- **Idaho Balsam Fir:** helps relieve headaches, stress, sore muscles and tension

- **Peppermint:** stimulates the mind and improves memory

- **Thieves oil**: helps relieve nasal congestion, stuffiness

- **Lemon**: acts as a natural antidepressant and calms anxiety

- **Orange**: refreshes and relaxes

- Basic air freshener: Simply add distilled water with 10-20 drops of your favorite oil and spray in any room. The spritzer can also be used for spraying your linens, bedding and towels.

- Use a cold-air oil diffuser. This is a great way to infuse your home with a continuous and subtle scent. Use Brain Power, Inspiration or Idaho Balsam Fir to especially activate the pineal, or choose Lemon, Lime or any of the citrus oils to help decalcify.

- Create your own potpourri: Use a crystal vase, china dish or wicker basket and add dried flower petals, pinecones or lavender florets. Then simply sprinkle your essential oil over it. Choose your oil according to what room you'd like to use this in. (see my Eco Green Your Holidays video on Rogers TV: http://www.rogerstv.com/page.aspx?lid=237&rid=51&gid=105025)

- Use rice as a potpourri: Fill a small decorative jar or dish with plain white rice and add in a few drops of oil. Place the jar in whatever room you wish to fill with the fragrance. I use peppermint or lemon for the bathroom and lavender for the bedroom.

- Create a hanging sachet with your essential oil of choice for activating the pineal. This is especially helpful in your office and bedroom. Add dried florets or pine cones to a mesh bag; add drops of your favorite pineal-stimulating essential oils.

- Infuse blotting paper or a clay pendant to hang in closets, laundry room and or bathrooms.

- Apply a few drops of lavender, or another calming essential oil, onto a cotton ball for your pillows. Place the cotton inside your pillowcase to help calm your senses as you drift off to sleep. Better still, add drops of one of the pineal activation oils- **Brain Power, Into The Future, or Inspiration or Blue Spruce**

- Dab cotton balls with essential oils and place in the corners of your drawers and closets. This tip not only helps with keeping clothes smelling fresh, but it also helps ward off moths!

Added tip: Use houseplants to detoxify and improve your air quality. A number of plants have been studied for their healthy air benefits. The *spider plant*, for example, was researched by NASA and found that it can reduce dangerous levels of toxins in a room by *96 percent in 24 hours.*

STEPS TO ELIMINATING MOLD

As discussed in my first Vibrational Cleaning book, and repeated here, mold can produce a variety of unhappy and even dangerous ailments. To eradicate and protect yourself from toxic mold, follow this regimen.

Remember: This is for 'What you can do'? This is an at Home Mold Cleaning method with essential oils.

If you suspect a leak or have major water problems make sure to contact a professional in your area.

What to Wear When Cleaning Moldy Areas

It is important to take precautions to **LIMIT YOUR EXPOSURE** to mold and mold spores.

1. Find if there is a leak or if there is a humidity problem first so that you can call in the experts to rectify this problem

2. **Use a mask:** In order to limit your exposure to airborne mold, you may want to wear an **N-95 respirator** (as recommended by the EPA). It is important to avoid breathing **in mold or mold spores. The respirator is** available at many hardware stores and from

companies that advertise on the Internet (They cost about $12 to $25.) The respirator or mask must fit properly to be effective, so carefully follow the instructions supplied with the respirator.

3. **Wear gloves:** Long gloves that extend to the middle of the forearm are recommended. When working with water and a mild detergent, ordinary household rubber gloves may be used. Avoid touching mold or moldy items with your bare hands.

4. **Wear goggles:** EPA recommends Goggles that do not have ventilation holes as a way to protect your eyes. Avoid getting mold or mold spores into your eyes.

Other Tips:

- Fix plumbing leaks and other water problems as soon as possible. Dry all items completely.

- Follow the 'Thieves Mold Removal' listed below before you begin the Mold cleanup.

- Absorbent or porous materials, such as ceiling tiles and carpet, clothing or furnishings may need to be thrown away if they become moldy. Make sure that these items are placed and sealed in an airtight plastic bag.

- Avoid exposing yourself or others to mold

- Do not paint or caulk moldy surfaces. Clean up the mold first and dry the surfaces before painting. Paint applied over moldy surfaces is likely to peel.

- If you are unsure about how to clean an item, or if the item is expensive or of sentimental value, you may wish to consult a specialist.

- Increase ventilation in closed areas such as bathrooms- (running a fan or opening a window) and cleaning more frequently will usually prevent mold from recurring, or at least keep the mold to a minimum.

OVERVIEW

Dr. Edward Close, an environmental engineer, environmental science expert and environmental advisor to Fortune 500 companies, whose work in eliminating mold with the use of Thieves essential oils highly recommends the method detailed below. [1, 2, 3]

#1. Diffuse Thieves essential oil, in a waterless or cold air diffuser, in the infested area and throughout the house. One 15ml bottle of Thieves will cover 1,000 square feet. You can run several diffusers at once.

Basic Non-Toxic Mold Removal

1. Sample first to determine the type of mold (toxic or non-toxic) that is present.

2. After samples have been collected, diffuse the Thieves Essential Oil Blend for 24 to 72 hours, non-stop in the space(s) where mold was found. Leave the room closed and sealed during this intensive diffusing.

3. Contact a professional to repair all leaks and eliminate all sources of moisture into the premises.

4. NO toxic mold after diffusing – clean visible mold with undiluted Thieves Household Cleaner, with gloves and mask.

5. Remove & seal any mold-infested materials in plastic & throw them away.

6. If toxic mold was found, then contact a professional for mold assistance.

#2. The more that the area is saturated with the aromatic compounds, the more effective the procedure will be. It is also important to use Thieves Household Cleaner to clean all areas, floor, ceilings, walls, bedding, countertops, etc. after diffusing.

MOLD PREVENTION

As a preventative, diffuse Thieves Essential Oil Blend for 8 hours continuously every week in your environment, or diffuse for 15 minutes every 3 hours. You'll be glad that you have.

THIEVES MOLD REMOVAL - STEPS

Eliminate mold and prevent it from returning!

CAUTION: If your home or space is saturated with mold, then contact a professional.

1. Sample first to determine the type of mold present (toxic or non-toxic). Toxic mold must be dealt with differently than non-toxic mold.

2. After samples have been collected,

69

3. **Diffuse the Thieves Essential Oil** Blend for 24 to 72 hours, non-stop, in the space(s) where mold was found. A cold-air diffuser, available via Young Living, works well in spaces up to 1000 sq. ft. in size. For best results, leave the room closed and sealed during this intensive diffusing. This will allow maximum penetration and absorption of the essential oil blend to inactivate the mold spores.

4. Contact a professional to repair all leaks and eliminate all sources of moisture into the premises.

5. If NO toxic mold was found, then after diffusing has been completed, **clean visible mold with undiluted Thieves Household Cleaner.** Use gloves, masks and other protective equipment. It is important to take precautions to avoid touching and breathing mold spores while cleaning.

6. Remove any mold-infested materials, seal them in plastic and throw them away.

7. If toxic mold was found, then contact a professional mold remediation service to have infested materials removed and to have them properly disposed of as these are hazardous materials. Diffuse in the sealed off space for 24 to 72 hours non-stop. Repairs must be done and infested materials replaced.

8. Have your professional resample to be sure all sources of mold have been identified and remediated. Repair all affected areas

9. If necessary, repeat the above steps 1 through 6, above.

10. Diffuse regularly for prevention and protection on a weekly basis or short periods each day.

MATERIALS NEEDED

- Thieves essential oil

- cold-air diffuser

- pail, mop and sponge

- rubber gloves

- protective mask- **N-95 respirator**

- Thieves Household Cleaner

CHAPTER 6

Green your deodorants!
Use common 'scents' under your arms

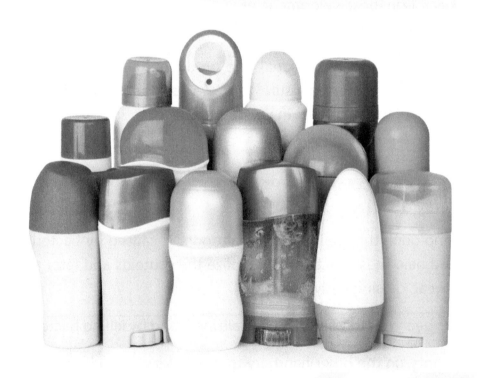

*"Only when the last tree has died and
The last river has been poisoned and
The last fish has been caught, Will we
realise that We cannot eat money"*

19th Century Cree Indian

STOP THE TOXIC DEODORANTS/ANTIPERSPIRANTS

Here is a reminder of some of the common major toxins found in deodorants that are discussed in more detail in the Vibrational Cleaning book. Then there are suggestions for replacing your deodorants below with essential oils.

- **Propylene Glycol** – used in anti-freeze, this chemical is implicated in contact dermatitis, kidney damage and liver abnormalities; can inhibit skin cell growth in human tests and can damage cell membranes causing rashes, dry skin and surface damage.

- **Triclosan** – Used as an antibacterial agent, this chemical has endocrine-disrupting properties amongst many other toxic effects. (See Chapter 1 in Vibrational Cleaning)

- **Parabens** – Known to have an estrogen-mimicking effect. Estrogen is well-known to play a key role in the development, growth and progression of breast cancer. (See Chapter 1 in Vibrational Cleaning)

Overall, topical applications of personal care products that contain parabens appear to be the greatest source of exposure to these estrogen-mimicking chemicals, far surpassing the risk of the aluminum in antiperspirants.

DEODORANT AND ANTIPERSPIRANT FACTS AS PRESENTED IN VIBRATIONAL CLEANING BOOK

- Sweat has no odor; the familiar unpleasant odor is caused by bacteria that live on our skin and hair. These bacteria metabolize the proteins and fatty acids from our apocrine sweat, causing body odor.

- Deodorants deal with the smell by neutralizing it and by killing bacteria.

- Antiperspirants, on the other hand, try to prevent sweating by blocking the pores using aluminum. Without sweat, the bacteria cannot metabolize proteins and fatty acids that cause body odor.

ANTIPERSPIRANTS: THE OVER-THE-COUNTER DRUG

You might be surprised to learn that the antiperspirant you use daily is in fact an over-the-counter (OTC) drug. As mentioned above, antiperspirants work by clogging, closing or blocking the pores with aluminum salts in order to prevent the release

of sweat, effectively changing the function of the body. Antiperspirants are considered to be drugs because they affect the physiology of the body.

Because antiperspirants are drugs, they are regulated by the Food and Drug Administration (FDA). Consequently, every antiperspirant sold in the US has a Drug Identification Number, which you can find on the label. A document called "monograph" states requirements for categories of non-prescription drugs such as antiperspirants. It defines, for example, what ingredients may be used and for what purpose. If the standards of the OTC monograph are met, premarket approval of a potentially new OTC product is not necessary.

Antiperspirants contain many active and inactive ingredients. Aluminum is the most common one. Most antiperspirants also contain paraben, an ingredient that is also used in deodorants.

THE NATURAL 'SCENTS-ABLE' SOLUTION

Your underarms are a very sensitive area: where your lymph area is located and responsible for the manufacturing of your white blood cells. Applying toxic deodorants or antiperspirants under your arms means that the toxins go directly into your lymphatic system! Instead, apply therapeutic, natural essential oils and receive the many benefits. Many essential oils can be applied directly under the armpits for effective protection, natural fragrance and herbal health benefits, along with the emotional and spiritual benefits. Essential oils are extremely effective at maintaining a normal underarm friendly 'aroma', but do not stop perspiration.

Listed below are some favorite solutions. Simply apply 3 to 5 drops of undiluted oil to your fingertips and rub it under each armpit as needed. The oils will do their job for 6 to 12 hours. Re-apply throughout the day when needed.

Not only does this method keep you somewhat dry, but the oils add benefits to harmonizing your system to improve your wellbeing.[2] If you need something stronger, then re-apply more often throughout the day. Another option is to use a readymade deodorant product like the Aroma Guard© natural deodorant available from Young Living that will keep you protected. You can check the website for more information for Aroma-Guard.

73

---

1. These statements have not been evaluated by the Food and Drug Administration. These products are not intended to diagnose, treat, cure, or prevent any disease.

REAL GREEN YOUR DEODORANTS

Please note Kosher Certification:

Many of Young Living Essential Oils's most popular products are also kosher-certified! Many of the oils listed below are Kosher certified. This means that a product is fit to use in any application in a manner that conforms to the kosher laws rooted in Biblical and Rabbinic traditions. Both the products and the facilities that produce them have been inspected and found to meet strict kosher requirements.

BERGAMOT ESSENTIAL OIL

- Used for hundreds of years for skin conditions especially for oily and troubled skin.

- It was trendy to use bergamot as a cologne and perfume during the Napoleonic era and is still used today to make perfumes.

- Bergamot (Citrus bergamia) has the fresh, sweet, citrus scent that is familiar to many as the flavoring in Earl Grey Tea. The scent is uplifting and relaxing, it is good for building confidence and enhancing your mood.

- Has many wellness properties that help maintain overall balance.

- Can be used for: Confidence, Calming and Female Hormonal Support

EUCALYPTUS GLOBULUS ESSENTIAL OIL

- Eucalyptus globulus has a fresh, penetrating scent. It contains a high percentage of the constituent eucalyptol, a key ingredient in many mouth rinses.

- Applied topically, it is often used to support the respiratory system and to soothe muscles after exercise and anytime for muscle tension

- Can be used for: respiratory support, muscle tension, skin support, deodorizer

According to Jean Valnet, MD a 2% solution of eucalyptus oil sprayed into the air will kill 70% of airborne staph bacteria.

LEMONGRASS ESSENTIAL OIL

- Lemongrass (Cymbopogon flexuosus) essential oil supports overall well-being and may support the digestive system. This oil contains the naturally occurring constituent geranial.

- Great support for healthy joints, ligaments, tendons and cartilage function

- Helpful in keeping unwanted insects at bay.

- Supports connective tissue function

- Use For: Purifying

- Used traditionally as a flavor enhancer by many cultures, adding Lemongrass oil is a delightful way to enhance the flavor of meals.

- Helps to balance the parasympathetic nervous system,

- Supports deep overall cleansing

- Lemongrass also protects our auric field from electromagnetic energy (TV, computers, radio).

***Can cause extreme skin irritation therefore, dilution is highly recommended if applied to the skin.

LEMON ESSENTIAL OIL

- Cold pressed from the fresh fruit peel of lemons grown in Argentina and the United States, lemon oil has refreshing and cooling properties.

- Its fresh, citrus scent is an instant pick-me-up.

- Supports the nervous, digestive and immune systems

- Has many wellness properties that help maintain overall balance.

- Calming plus many other relaxing benefits

- It is widely used in all types of skin care for cleansing the skin and helping to promote younger, fresher looking skin.

- It is cleansing to the spiritual bodies as well as to the liver and kidney systems

ROSEMARY ESSENTIAL OIL

- Rosemary essential oil helps support a healthy lifestyle regimen and overall wellness.

- This oil provides a savory addition to many meals such as meats, marinades, side dishes, and dressings.

- Rosemary includes the naturally occurring constituents' eucalyptol and alpha-pinene.

- Can use for: mental clarity and liver support, lung support, healthy skin maintainence.

- Supports healthy hair growth, and a healthy immune system.

- Keeps the mind alert and focused.

CYPRESS ESSENTIAL OIL

- Cypress (Cupressus sempervirens) is especially comforting during the winter season.

- Cypress is beneficial for circulation and supports a healthy flowing lymph system

- The fragrance is relaxing for emotional trauma, calming & soothing for angry feelings

- Its fresh, herbaceous, slightly evergreen aroma is refreshing and restores feelings of security and stability.

- Cypress is also beneficial for oily or troubled skin.

GENTLE BABY ESSENTIAL OIL BLEND

- Gentle Baby™ is a soft, fragrant combination of essential oils designed specifically for mothers and babies. Gentle Baby contains quite an assortment of essential oils that are used in elite cosmetics to enhance a youthful appearance. (Contains: Pelargonium graveolens† (Geranium) flower oil, Aniba rosaeodora† (Rosewood) wood oil, Coriandrum sativum† (Coriander) seed oil, Cymbopogon martini† (Palmarosa) oil, Lavandula angustifolia† (Lavender) oil, Cananga odorata† (Ylang

ylang) flower oil, Anthemis nobilis† (Roman chamomile) flower oil, Citrus limon† (Lemon) peel oil, Jasminum officinale** (Jasmine) oil, Rosa damascena† (Rose) flower oil

- It helps calm emotions during pregnancy and is useful for quieting troubled little ones.

- The fragrance is relaxing and balancing, helping to restore confidence and reduce stress.

- It is also soothing to tender and revitalizing for dry skin.

GERANIUM ESSENTIAL OIL

- The fragrance is relaxing and balancing.

- The fragrance also helps release negative memories and balance nervous tension and frustration.

- Geranium (Pelargonium graveolens) has a wonderfully uplifting, calming, flowery scent.

- It is also soothing to the skin and revitalizing for dry skin.

- Its aromatic influence helps release negative memories.

- Used traditionally to support the circulatory and nervous systems, a great deal of its strength lies in its ability to revitalize body tissues.

- Supports healthy digestive system, Respiratory Support and Liver Support.

- Can be used for Women's Health.

LAVENDER ESSENTIAL OIL

- Steam distilled from the flowering plants grown at the Young Living farms in Simiane-la-Rotonde, France, and Mona, Utah, lavender is the most versatile essential oil.

- Use For: skin irritations, balancing and relaxation

- Its refreshing, relaxing scent has balancing properties that also brings a sense of calm, helping to increase cognitive performance.

- Supports restful sleep.

Use for promoting younger, fresher looking skin.

PALMAROSA ESSENTIAL OIL

- Palmarosa (Cymbopogon martini) essential oil is steam distilled from the leaves of the plant.

- This oil can be stimulating and soothing to the body and mind. Good for cellular support and skin health

- Aromatherapists love Palmarosa for its skin conditioning properties, its calming, floral scent.

- Fragrance creates a feeling of security, balance, reduces stress and tension.

- Promotes a healthy and speedy recovery from exhaustion.

- Palmarosa was added to Indian curry dishes and West African meat dishes to destroy bacteria and aid digestion.

PATCHOULI ESSENTIAL OIL

- Patchouli essential oil may improve the appearance of dry, chapped skin and is an ideal complement when added to your favorite skin care products.

- Diffuse this oil for a calming, relaxing, peaceful fragrance.

- Helps to clarify thoughts and balance emotional feelings

- Use For: Skin Health, Emotional Release, and Anti-nausea Support

ROYAL HAWAIIAN SANDALWOOD ESSENTIAL OIL

- Royal Hawaiian Sandalwood (Santalum paniculatum) has a rich, sweet, warm, and woody aroma that is sensual and romantic.

- The S. paniculatum tree is native to and found only on the island of Hawaii, where Young Living has a partner farm that practices sustainable reforestation farming management principles.

- Used traditionally as incense in religious ceremonies and for meditation, this oil is uplifting and relaxing.

- It is grounding and stabilizing.

- Fragrance helps to remove negative programming from the cells, stimulating for the pineal gland.

- It is valued in skin care for its moisturizing and normalizing properties.

VETIVER ESSENTIAL OIL

- Vetiver (Vetiveria zizanoides) has a heavy, earthy fragrance similar to patchouli with a touch of lemon that men may like to use for skin care.

- Vetiver oil is psychologically grounding, calming, relaxing and stabilizing.

- One of the oils that is highest in sesquiterpenes, vetiver was studied by Dr. Terry Friedmann for improving children's behavior.

- Vetiver may help when coping with stress and to recover from emotional trauma and shock. Emotional Grounding

- Sleep Support

YLANG YLANG ESSENTIAL OIL

- **Ylang Ylang essential oil has a rich, sweet, floral scent that is pleasing and romantic and can be diffused to create a calming, relaxing and soothing atmosphere.**

- **Used for skin care and supports cardio-vascular system.**

- **Fragrance helps to balance male /female energies and uplifts low self-esteem**

- **Massage into the scalp to increase the appearance of healthy, shiny hair.**

CHAPTER 7

Insect 'Scents' Makes Sense

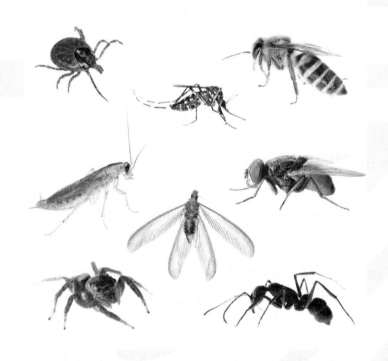

"To keep the body in good health is a duty... otherwise we shall not be able to keep our mind strong and clear."

Buddha

SCENTSABLE ACTION

Now you can take scents-able action with
Real Green Essentials© for unwanted pests.

Anytime one spends time outdoors, pesky insects can make one's experience most unpleasant with stings and bites. Stings often result in redness and swelling in the injured area. Sometimes a sting can cause a life-threatening allergic reaction. **Considering both multiple stings and allergic reactions to single stings, insects actually harm or even kill (in rare cases) more than three times as many North Americans as snakes do. Scientists estimate** that between one and two million people worldwide die each year mainly from malaria, the most common of the mosquito-borne illnesses. Obviously, insect bites can be a quick way to destroy one's life or make one's life more challenging or miserable.

Approximately, one in five people are especially attractive for mosquitoes to feast on. You certainly don't want to be one of them. Roughly 200 out of the 3,000 species of mosquitoes in the world can be found in the US. Not only is it important to protect yourself from the bites but it's also critical to lessen your likelihood of contracting any of the well-known mosquito-borne illnesses, such as malaria, or any of the other mosquito-borne illnesses, like encephalitis, yellow fever, West Nile virus or dengue. One interesting fact about mosquitoes:

- **Mosquitoes actually feed on plant nectars. It's the female mosquitoes that use blood to nourish their eggs prior to laying, imbibing about 5 millionths of a liter per "feeding." (Dr. Mercola 1)**

Tips and natural formulas are given below to help you avoid the pesticides as insect repellents. As an overview, remember that there are so many dangers to using DEET (N,N-diethyl-m-toluamide) – the most widely used repellent. **DEET is a registered pesticide. It is a member of the toluene chemical family which is a hazardous waste and an endocrine disruptor as well as a potential cancer causing agent.**

DEET can cause severe skin irritation, blistering and burning in some individuals and interfere with your nervous system. Most often, DEET is used with other pesticides, creating highly dangerous combinations. One of these is permethrin. Permethrin in itself is quite toxic and especially to cats. It is a member of the synthetic pyrethroid family, known as a neurotoxin (which means it will be damaging to the pineal and pituitary glands). **The EPA has even classified this chemical carcinogenic: It causes lung tumors, liver tumors, immune system problems and chromosomal abnormalities.**

Mosquitoes **can at least temporarily overcome or adapt to the repellent effect of DEET after an initial exposure**, representing a non-genetic behavioral change. Sadly, DEET is still widely used. According to the EPA, every year, approximately **one-third** of the U.S. population is expected to use DEET.

It is best to avoid any harmful chemical repellent that is sold on the market and instead make your own Real Green bug protection.

MOTHER NATURE'S KEYS TO DETER MOSQUITOES
GREEN THUMBS TO ESSENTIAL OILS

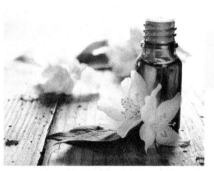

This section is worth repeating as it is fully explained in my Vibrational Cleaning book. Two botanical repellents which performed particularly well in a Florida study as a repellent were lemon eucalyptus essential oil (providing 120 minutes of protection) and Citronella oil (30-40 minutes of protection). The authors note that the oils just need to be applied more often.

Lemon eucalyptus oil also known **as *Eucalyptus citriadora* provides protection similar to repellents with low concentrations of DEET as reported by the CDC.** The CDC has given its approval for **lemon eucalyptus as an effective repellent**.

Neem oil blended with coconut or jojoba oil is another plant-based traditional Indian insect repellent. **Catnip and thyme essential oils** were found to be more effective in warding off mosquitoes and other bugs than DEET.

Dr. Joseph Mercola reported another study that showed cinnamaldehyde, the chief constituent found in **cinnamon leaf oil,** to be effective as a pesticide—without the risk of

83

negative health and environmental consequences. A pest-control company in Spokane Valley, Washington, published a study[1] in the industry journal *Pest Management Science* about testing the potential repellency of essential oils against yellow jackets (mainly *Vespula pensylvanica*) and paper wasps (mainly *Polistes dominulus*). Two essential oil blends, one with three essential oils, **clove, geranium, and lemongrass**, and one with a four-oil blend of **clove, geranium, lemongrass and rosemary** showed significant repellency. Both blends "totally blocked the attraction of vespid workers."[2]

Essential oils are the active ingredient in many brand-name products. Of course, using the real natural product that is unhampered by chemical solvents and the like is the best alternative, giving you the most in usage and safety. Just a reminder: There are many essential oil companies. Not all essential oils are created equal. Purity and quality is absolutely critical in order to obtain maximum results and safety.

My choice (as explained earlier) is the use of a therapeutic, genuine; clean, all organic essential oil by Young Living Company. It is recognized today as the world leader in genuine, pure and edible essential oils, producing the highest quality on the market.

In Summary some potent, effective and safe uses of essential oils:

- Cinnamon leaf oil is effective as a pesticide (found in one study to be more effective at killing mosquitoes than DEET)

- Citronella oil use as a wash- mix a few drops of citronella in a spray bottle and spray arms, neck and legs - used all over the world for thousands of years as an insect repellent!

- **Some of the Plant Properties:** Antibacterial, antioxidant, antifungal, anti-inflammatory, antiseptic, antiparasitic, antispasmodic, deodorant, insecticidal and relaxant.

- Catnip oil (according to one study, this oil is 10 times more effective than DEET)

- Lemon eucalyptus was found very effective in a 2014 Australian study; a mixture of 32 percent lemon eucalyptus oil provided more than 95 percent protection for three hours, compared to a 40 percent DEET repellent that gave 100 percent protection for seven hours

- As recommended in a June 2014 article on AlterNet, use a natural formula that contains a combination of citronella, lemongrass oil, peppermint oil and vanillin to repel mosquitoes, fleas, chiggers, ticks and other biting insects.

What insects cause itchy or painful bites?

Mosquito bites, harvest mites (also called chiggers), fleas, and bedbugs usually cause itchy, red bumps. The size of the swelling can vary from a dot to a centimetre (half inch). Mosquito bites near the eye usually cause serious swelling for multiple days.

Clues that a bite is a mosquito bite are itchiness, a central raised dot in the swelling, and presence of the bite on a surface not covered by clothing. Some mosquito bites in sensitive children form hard lumps that last for months. In contrast to mosquitoes, fleas and bedbugs don't fly; therefore, they crawl under clothing to nibble. Flea bites often turn into little blisters in young children.

Bites of horseflies, deerflies, gnats, fire ants, harvester ants, blister beetles, and centipedes usually cause a painful, red bump. Within a few hours, fire ant bites change to blisters or pimples.

More bug-safety ideas:

- Eliminate breeding grounds by removing sources of standing water (flowerpots, kiddie pools, garbage bins, birdbaths, etc.)

- Use yellow outdoor light bulbs to help reduce mosquito populations at night.

- Use a fan when there is little wind, since mosquitoes are not strong flyers and the wind disturbs the chemical sweat coming off your bodies.

- Plant mosquito-repelling plants like lemon balm, catnip, basil and lemon geraniums around outdoor sitting areas.

- Encourage mosquito predators like bats, dragonflies, birds, frogs and beetles, which can help reduce mosquito populations.

- Mosquitoes are also attracted by carbon dioxide, lactic acid and other body chemicals, as well as your body heat and sweat, and can sense these chemicals from 25-35 meters. Larger people naturally emit more carbon dioxide than smaller people, which is one of the reasons adults seem to be bitten more often than children.

- Be aware beer drinking increases carbon dioxide. Women and people drinking beer have been shown to be more attractive to mosquitoes. That makes women who drink beer more vulnerable!

- Blonds seem to be favored as well by mosquitoes compared to brunettes.

- In one study, a full moon increased mosquito activity by 500 percent. (Mercola)

- Use essential oils either singularly or any formula mix below prior to your outings, this will help avoid the need for any chemical repellent.

DETER INSECT SPRAYS AND BUG BITE SOOTHERS

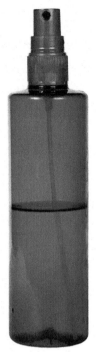

Make your own homemade insect sprays and lotions and soothe those annoying bug bites without chemicals.

• As a general rule, use *Lemongrass or Citronella* to keep insects at bay: Diffuse into the air, infuse paper strips at the windows, on light bulbs, etc.

• Use **lavender** oil to deter insects from landing on your skin.

• Olive oil is in itself an insect repellent. So mix 5 tablespoons **olive oil** with equal amounts of *cinnamon oil* (a powerful repellent) and mix it well. Will keep mosquitoes away from you.

• Dab oils neat on neck and legs, or use a spray bottle.

• Ankles are a prime target for mosquitoes. Cover the ankles with cotton socks and add a drop of **Lavender or Purification** to the tops of the socks. Put drops of essential oils on bottom of pant legs.

All-purpose insect spray and lotion:

To make a spray, use a base of witch hazel, olive oil, or vodka. Add one or a combination of the oils listed below, at a ratio of 10 parts base to 2 parts essential oil. Mix in a spray bottle.

• **Lemongrass**

• **Eucalyptus citriadora (most effective)**

• **Thyme**

• **Peppermint**

• **Lavender**

• **Cinnamon**

• **Cedarwood**

• **Palo Santo**

- **Citronella (most effective)**

- **Purification Blend (most effective)**

To make a lotion, add 120 drops of the above listed oils to two ounces of distilled water in a deep mixing bowl. Using a wire whip, beat the mixture quickly while gradually adding two ounces of olive oil. Store the mixture in a jar or bottle and use as needed. Especially useful while hiking.

Insect Deterrent

- Combine **4 drops Thyme, 8 drops Lemongrass, 4 drops Lavender, 4 drops Peppermint, 8 drops Lemon Eucalyptus and 4 drops Cinnamon oil**. Mix together and apply neat, or add to a 8-ounce bottle with distilled water.

House and garden bug spray - Green Pesticides

- 3 drops of **Spearmint and 3 drops Orange oil** mixed in 2 quarts water. Spray on plants in the house and outside to keep the bugs and aphids away.

- Mix equal parts of vinegar with a cap of Thieves Household Cleaner concentrate in a quart of water. Spray on plants.

- **Preparation for another natural- green pesticide**

- Fill an 8-oz. spray bottle with distilled water

- Add 1 ½ tablespoons of liquid dish soap- preferably Thieves household cleaner

- Add 3–4 drops of each of the oils listed below:

- Spearmint essential oil,

- Citronella essential oil

- Lavender essential oil

- Blue tansy essential oil

- Cedarwood essential oil essential oil

- Mix and spray generously on plants, fruits, and vegetables

- – Thanks to Marco Colindres III, YL Product Marketing Manager for the above recipe listed on the Young Living website.

- Spearmint essential oil can help deter ants and aphids

- Citronella essential oil can help deter gnats and mosquitoes

- Lavender essential oil can help deter fleas, moths and flies

- Blue tansy essential oil can help deter flies

- Cedarwood essential oil can help deter snails and slugs

Fungus on plants:

Lemon and orange essential oils can help reduce fungi from growing on plants- by simply adding 3-4 drops to a 8 oz bottle of water.

Mosquito Spray

- Combine in equal parts: Citronella, *Eucalyptus citriadora* (Lemon Eucalyptus), Basil, Lemongrass, Thyme, Patchouli and Cinnamon oil.

- Combine Lemon, Peppermint, Eucalyptus, Lemongrass and Citronella.

- Young Living Oil Blends: Lemongrass with Citronella, Idaho Tansy with floral water, Purification, Thieves or Melrose.

Oils for other insects

- Moth Deterrent: Patchouli

- Horse-Fly deterrent: Idaho tansy (create floral water and spray)

- Aphid deterrent: Mix 10 drops spearmint and 15 drops orange essential oils in 2 quarts salt water. Shake well and spray on plants.

- Cockroach deterrent: Mix 10 drops peppermint and 5 drops cypress in ½ cup salt water. Shake well and spray where roaches live.

- Silverfish deterrent: Eucalyptus radiata, Eucalyptus citriadora

STINK MOSQUITOES AWAY THROUGH DIET

Mosquitoes are attracted to body odor and sweat so making your sweat unattractive to them can be done through your diet. People eating diets rich in whole grains, fruits and vegetables have noted that they receive fewer mosquito bites than those consuming more processed and sugary foods. Forgo bananas during mosquito season, as something about how they are metabolized appears to attract mosquitoes. Changing your diet could potentially provide the simplest way to repel mosquitoes naturally.

It's been found that vitamin B-1 or thiamine alters your human scent. An earlier study in the 1960s, though inconclusive, indicated that taking vitamin B1 (thiamine) may be effective in discouraging mosquitoes from biting. The theory is based on the premise that taking more vitamin B1 than your body requires causes the excess to be excreted through your urine, skin, and sweat. The skin odor produced by vitamin B-1 seems to be offensive to the female mosquitoes. This may account for the popularity of brewer's yeast as a mosquito repellent, since it's high in thiamine.

Some research suggests that regular consumption of garlic or garlic capsules may help protect against both mosquito and tick bites.

NATURAL SUPPORT FOR BITES AND STINGS WITH NATURAL AGENTS

Once you've been bitten, then the objective is to treat the bite or sting immediately. There are a variety of ways to soothe the skin with natural agents and essential oils that have balancing properties.

- Reduce irritation by making your own lavender-peppermint spray: To one cup distilled water, add **20 drops lavender and 20 drops peppermint oils**. This will help to reduce bite-induced itching and infection.

- Disinfect bites by combining **10 drops Lavender with 20 drops Thyme and 10 drops Lemon Eucalyptus. Or** add **8 drops each of these oils, with 5 drops Oregano**, to a bowl of water or spray bottle filled with water for washing the skin.

- Use a blend called Purification that is made up of citronella, lemongrass, lavandin, rosemary, melaleuca, and myrtle. It helps to reduce the swelling and to neutralize the poisons.

- **Basil oil** can also be used to soothe or reduce the swelling and is known to neutralize poisons.

- Take a few drops of **Oregano, Longevity or Exodus oils (special Young Living blends) internally** several times throughout the day with water. Or take 2-4 **Longevity** capsules (a Young Living supplement) a day as well. Take **Sulferzyme** (special blend of methylsulfonylmethane (MSM) and Wolfberry) 6- 12 capsules a day help support the body's natural immunity to reduce swelling and itchiness.

- Here's another recipe to use as a remedy for insect bites... mix and apply

  - ✓ 2 drops **thyme**

  - ✓ 10 drops **lavender**

  - ✓ 4 drops **eucalyptus radiata**

  - ✓ 3 drops **German chamomile**

VIRTUES OF LAVENDER ESSENTIAL OIL

Lavender has been used for over 2,500 years.

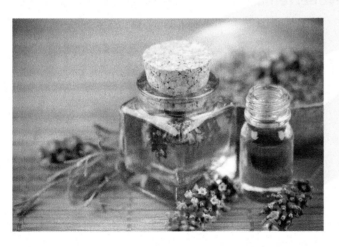

Throughout history, lavender was used for various purposes. The Phoenicians, Arabians, and Egyptians used lavender as a perfume, as well as for mummification, they simply wrapped the mummies with lavender-dipped garments. Later in Greece and Rome, it was used as an all-around cure. In Medieval and Renaissance Europe, it was scattered all over stone castle floors as a natural disinfectant and deodorant. Lavender was rediscovered for its healing properties by Dr. Gattefossé, a French bio-chemist in the 1920's.

Lavender has many Plant Properties: Antifungal, analgesic, antiseptic, antitumoral, anticonvulsant, vasodilating, antispasmodic, anti-inflammatory, vermifuge, insecticidal.

91

BENEFITS OF LAVENDER OIL

Used for Stress and balancing many body systems to support and maintain a healthy immune system.

Lavender helps with memory formation and to maintain focus.

These particular beneficial properties of lavender are suitable in both preventing insect bites and soothing insect bites and stings. Lavender oil has been used as a bug repellent and for soothing insect bites for many centuries. Lavender flowers were used in the past to protect clothes and linens from the infestation of moths and other insects as well as to keep the clothing smelling fresh.

Lavender oil helps to prevent the spread of infection caused by a bug bite as well as controlling the itching and inflammation often associated with bug bites. Author, aroma therapist, Valerie Ann Worwood, writes in her book "The Complete Book of Essential Oils and Aromatherapy," that lavender oil is an aid to controlling the infestation of fleas, black fly, black beetle, flies, greenfly and white fly.

BEE STING FIRST AID TREATMENTS

1. **If the bee that stung you was a honeybee, remove the stinger as soon as possible, use your fingers if need be.**

2. **Look for symptoms of an allergic reaction to the sting as listed below:**

- Difficulty breathing

- Hives that appear as a red, itchy rash and spread to areas beyond the sting

- Swelling of the face, throat or mouth tissue

- Wheezing or difficulty swallowing

- Restlessness and anxiety

- Rapid pulse

- Dizziness or a sharp drop in blood pressure

- • If the symptoms are present, seek emergency medical attention immediately!

Take an antihistamine as soon as possible (support the body's immunity as well with several drops such as lavender oil every 10- 15 minutes or supplement Sulferzyme)

- If need be use the epinephrine part of an emergency allergy kit, your Epipen, if it has been prescribed in the past. (**http://www.webmd.com/allergies/guide/insect-stings**)

ESSENTIAL OILS TO APPLY IMMEDIATELY

Single oils: apply on location either **Lavender or Idaho Tansy**. Can also apply any of these special Young Living blends: **Purification**, Melrose, or Pan Away on area of concern.

Bee Sting Blends

- Mix 2 drops Lavender, 1 drop Helichrysum, 1 drop Chamomile, 1 drop Wintergreen- apply to the sting several times throughout the day.

- Or mix and apply 1 or 2 drops Purification, Melrose, Lavender, or Idaho Tansy on location. Repeat until the venom spread has stopped.

- Or mix and apply 2 drops lavender, 1 drop German chamomile and 1 drop wintergreen.

- Apply Lavender with or without one or more of the single oils listed, 2 to 3 times daily or every hour until redness abates. Apply 1-2 drops of one of the Bee Sting Blends on the location every 15 minutes for the first hour.

Other Supportive steps:

1. Flick or scrape stinger out with credit card or pin, taking care not to squeeze the venom sack. Or mix baking soda with several drops of lavender oil and water- apply the paste to the area and let dry. This will help to pull out the venom if applied immediately and works quickly to help balance your immunity.

2. Apply ice wrapped in fabric to the bee sting for 20 minutes to alleviate the swelling and the pain.

3. Apply the special Young Living Thieves toothpaste on the bee sting as it contains a special blend of essential oils that will help. The cool feeling is also relieving.

Hornets, Wasps and Yellow Jackets

Some of the most painful stings come not from bees, but hornets, wasps, or yellow jackets.

These stinging insects are all part of the family *Vespidae*. Members of the wasp family also do not leave stingers in their victims, as do bees.

Use the same oil blends as for bees to soothe the sting as much as possible as you seek medical attention.

Chigger (Mite) Bites

- **Use Lavender, Tea tree (melaleuca) or Purification or Melrose blend. Massage 2 to 6 drops of undiluted oil on location, 3-5 times daily.**

Ticks

- **Apply the essential oil (Purification, Thyme or Oregano oil) immediately to prevent the tick from embedding deeper into the skin.**

- **Use any of these oils: single oils of Thyme, Oregano, Peppermint, RC Blend or Purification blend.**

- **Apply Thyme oil to tick to loosen from skin. Then apply Purification on site to detoxify wound and to also loosen the tick- often times the tick will back out from the skin after applying this oil blend.**

- **Apply 1 drop Peppermint every 5 minutes for 50 minutes to reduce pain and infection.**

- **Take Oregano capsules internally throughout the day as well as Longevity capsules to help boost your immune system.**

Brown Recluse Spider Bite:

The bite of this spider causes painful redness and blistering which progresses to a gangrenous slough of the affected area. **Seek immediate medical attention** and use this treatment in the interim.

- **Spider bite blend: 1 drop Lavandin, 1 drop Helichrysum, 1 drop Melrose—or use Purification Blend. Apply one drop of either of the 2 above blends until reaching medical treatment.**

BED Bugs! Spray them away the real green way!

Who wants to share their bed with these pesky critters- it certainly isn't a comforting thought. Instead share your bed with the Thieves essential oil blend.

Thieves Bug Spray #1

- **Thieves® Spray bottle**

- **6 drops Clove, Eucalyptus or Melaleuca essential oil**

- **6 drops of a citrus essential oil such as Lemon, Lime, Orange, Bergamot or Citrus Fresh**

Add Clove (or other) essential oil and your choice of your favourite citrus essential oil directly into the Thieves Spray bottle. Shake well and spray.

This is an easy formula to use for hotel beds.

 At home, wash your bedding in Thieves household cleaner with the addition of Citrus Fresh or Lemon, Lime, Bergamot essential oils.

Tip: When traveling and want to avoid bringing home any bed bugs, make a sachet to place in your suitcase by spraying on the Thieves Bug Spray on either a cotton ball or washcloth.

Thieves Bug Spray #2

- **Add these oils to a spray bottle, filled with 4 ounces of distilled water.**

- **20 drops Thieves essential oil blend**

- **10 drops of either Lemon, Lime, Bergamot, Orange, or Citrus Fresh**

- **4 drops Clove essential oil**

- **10 drops Eucalyptus Globulus**

Shake vigorously before using. Make sure to spray in all areas around your bed –the bed frame, mattress and flooring. Spray the sheets as well as washing the sheets in the same mixture by adding the formula to your wash load.

Sun baked skin? Use Lava Derm Cooling Mist -

Bring relief to stressed skin with a blend of gentle skin-soothing ingredients that include lavender essential oil mixed with Aloe Vera. Spray directly onto the affected area and repeat every 10-15 minutes until desired relief is achieved.

Contains: Deionized Water, Aloe Barbadensis (Aloe Vera) Leaf Concentrate, Lavandula Angustifolia† (Lavender) Oil, and Ionic Trace Minerals.

NATURAL INSECT CHART

GREEN BUG SPRAYS QUICK GUIDE

For more specific insect problems, try mixing 8 ounces of water in a spray bottle with ½ tsp. of natural Thieves soap and 12 drops of Young Living essential oil from the guide below. Remember to shake the bottle frequently to keep the oil mixed with the water!

Ants	Peppermint (add a line to window and door seals)
Aphids	Peppermint, sandalwood, white fir
Beetles	Peppermint, thyme
Caterpillars	Peppermint
Chiggers	Lavender, lemongrass, thyme
Cutworm	Thyme
Fleas	Lavender, lemongrass, peppermint
Flies	Basil, clove, eucalyptus, lavender, peppermint, rosemary
Gnats	Patchouli
Mosquitoes	Lavender, lemongrass, Purification, Palo Santo
Moths	Lavender, peppermint
Plant Lice	Peppermint
Roaches	Eucalyptus
Slugs	White fir
Snails	Patchouli, white fir
Spiders	Peppermint
Ticks	Lavender, lemongrass, thyme
Weevils	Patchouli, sandalwood

TREATMENT QUICK GUIDE
NATURAL QUICK HOME GUIDE TIPS

ESSENTIAL OIL	HERBAL	OTHER
Lavender oil is one of the most versatile and popular essential oils for its calming scent, and antimicrobial and protective insect properties.	Tea bags: Cool a tea bag and swipe it over your bites. The tannins in the tea act as an astringent, to reduce swelling.	Cucumbers: Cool as a cucumber- and it is helpful for reducing swelling and the heat.
Cinnamon oil can deter mosquitoes, and has been well researched for its antibacterial and antifungal properties as well.	Chamomile tea: is a very soothing herb that can be applied to the skin with a wet tea bag or the essential oil.	
Basil oil contains camphor and thymol, two compounds that can relieve itching. It is also able to neutralize the poisons. Apply directly to the bite.	Aloe Vera: Contains more than 130 active compounds and 34 amino acids that are beneficial to your skin.	Baking soda- Dissolve in your bath water mixed with lavender or chamomile essential oil and soak for 30 minutes.
Palo Santo Oil or "Holy Wood" is **rare** and **unique** oil from Ecuador. And the indigenous people in South America have used it for thousands of years for its powerful healing properties. Also used in South America to repel mosquitoes, for fevers, infections and skin diseases.		Witch hazel: Make a paste out of witch hazel and baking soda with a few drops of lavender or citronella or chamomile and apply directly to your bite to reduce swelling.
Peppermint oil is cooling and can help to bring balance and relief to pain, itching, heat and provide temporary relief.		Apple cider vinegar: Can be added to your bath to help relieve itching. Add two to three cups to your bath and soak for 30 minutes.
Tea Tree oil: Helpful for healing cuts, dis-infecting and soothing to bites.		
Citronella essential oil It is a natural mosquito repellent that performed well in a Florida study. It is also a natural antifungal; so can include it in blends for skin fungus.		

CHAPTER 8

Pineal Exposed
Review and More Notes

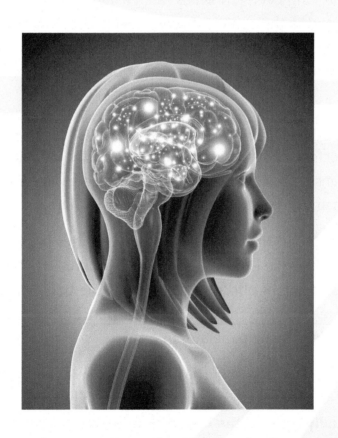

*"Keep the Pineal Gland Operating
and You Won't Grow Old - You Will
Always be Young."*

- Edgar Cayce

WHY THE PINEAL GLAND?

Over many years, I observed the energetic state of the mysterious pineal gland amongst my clients by using my GDV Kirlian camera, an advanced bio-electrography device that accurately measures the body's energy fields. The pineal gland is considered to be the key to the universe, a pea-sized gland that lies deep within the center of the human brain behind the pituitary gland. It has been a mystery for nearly two thousand years.

Many people don't know how important this gland is! In recent years, findings in neurochemistry and anthropology have given greater credence to the folklore that **the pineal gland is the 'third eye', source of 'second sight', 'seat of the soul', or the psychic centre within the brain.** It is considered to be our mind's eye and is the reason why we DREAM.

The pineal gland has long been known as the master gland or the gland that governs over our third eye and is the center of psychic awareness in the human mind. This amazing gland produces a hormone we may have heard about, called melatonin which regulates human daily body rhythms that deal directly with the day and night cycles.

Developing and expanding the function and the energy of our pineal gland is extremely important as it affects every physical bodily system. The pineal has the potential to determine the expansion or contraction of our psychic awareness, our consciousness, our intuition, our memory and our experience with the Divine.

Current research has found that the pineal is a very active organ, having the **second highest blood flow** after the kidneys and equal in volume to the pituitary. The pineal has the highest absorption of phosphorus in the whole body and the **second highest absorption of iodine,** after the thyroid. No other part of the brain contains so much serotonin or is capable of making melatonin.

The pineal gland is unique in the body: It is an unpaired midline organ in the brain which has resisted encroachment by the corpus callosum. Whilst being right in the centre of the brain, **it is actually outside the blood-brain barrier and so is theoretically not part of the brain!**

In Hindu traditions, the pineal gland is associated with our extra-sensory third 'eye' through which perception of the world is not limited to the physical senses. In Native American traditions, it's associated with the 'vision quest.'

Every emotion we feel, every moment of joy and fear, produces a chemical enzyme in our body. Each enzyme passes through to the pineal. The pineal is the system of entry into the Divine Mind. It is a complex crystalline computer that screens frequencies both with thoughts and feelings.

In the ancient Vedic energy system of the chakras, the pineal gland is referred to as **'Ajna' or '3rd Eye' chakra.** It is a well known symbol in Eastern literature. The ancients considered the pineal as a very important organ and knew that, in fact, the pineal gland functions very much like an eye, an inner eye- **the 'third eye'.**

Mathew, King James Version, verse 6, summarized the importance of the pineal by stating:

"The light of the body is the eye, if therefore thine eye be single, thy whole body shall be full of light."

Fill the pineal with light and the whole body shall be full of light. What's interesting to note: Essential oils are captured light in molecules and vapors.

René Descartes (1596-1650) was one of the early philosophers who attached great significance to the pineal gland. He was experienced in vivisection and anatomy and he regarded the pineal as the *'principal seat of the soul'*- the meeting place of the physical and the spiritual. He rightly pointed out the unique nature of the pineal gland's location in the brain being located near the center of the brain, between the two hemispheres but outside the protection of the blood-brain barrier. Exposed to a high volume of blood flow, the pineal gland is quite vulnerable to chemical toxins.

MYSTERIES OF THE PINEAL GLAND REVEALED

Modern studies reveal that the gland's watery interior contains rods and cones-just like those found in the retina of our eyes! This means that our '3rd eye' has a structure remarkably similar to our two physical eyes. This is why when we visualize something strongly enough, we can literally see it "in our mind's eye". The Pineal Gland acts as the **interface between the higher dimensions and the physical realm** –just like Descartes had mapped out earlier. Psychics consider it to be the link for *inter dimensional experiences* and **a Portal to the Divine** so that our higher light and unconditional love can enter into our physical form.

The pineal is our inter-dimensional doorway to higher consciousness and bliss and facilitates multidimensional thinking, mastery of energy and manifestation via thought waves amongst many other functions.

In the Ancient Spiritual Mystery Schools, they knew the real importance of the Pineal Gland and found ways to stimulate it into its magnificent and final role of transforming consciousness and Awakening. Now, today, we too can activate the Pineal Gland and dramatically accelerate our Spiritual Path to Awakening. When the Pineal Gland is fully activated it assists us in **consciously accessing the 95 % of the brain that scientists say is unused**. These areas of the brain are referred to as *the Sacred Chambers and contain our spiritual gifts,* expanded abilities, Universal Knowledge and connection with our Divine Source.

With a fully activated Pineal, its influence will assist us in many areas of our life. It will help bring our life into alignment with our life purpose and mission, assist with the transformation of our mind and emotions, expand our consciousness and activate all strands of our DNA. In addition to this rapid expansion of consciousness, many people also find they begin to quickly resolve issues in their life such as relationship, work, health, finances, etc. This activation and awakening assists in the transformation of our Being on many levels including physical, mental, emotional and Spiritual.

ARE WE BLOCKING OUR INTER-DIMENSIONAL DOORWAY? OUR HYPER - GATEWAY TO HIGHER DIMENSIONS?

The Pineal obviously plays an important role in our overall well-being: Unfortunately for most of us, this gland is *atrophied, dormant and* **calcified** to the point of *being useless*. Neuro-toxic chemicals poison our pineal and the most common ones are found in our own homes as household and personal care products. A number of these are outlined in detail in Chapter 1 in my **"Vibrational Cleaning"** book. *Our household cleaners, laundry detergents, soaps, perfumes and fluoride all block the function of our third eye. Even if we changed these toxic products, none on the market place have products that can detox and activate our pineal at the same time - but we can with these authentic, clean, pure essential oils!*

One of the most toxic chemicals to the pineal is **FLUORIDE!** Fluoride will calcify this gland and render it dormant by the time we are a teenager. If you and I are looking to become spiritually aware, then this is the gland we want to have fully functioning…the "seat of the soul".

During the late 1990's, Jennifer Luke, a scientist in England at the University of Surrey, determined that the pineal gland, located in the middle of the brain, was a target for fluoride-. She undertook the first study of the effects of sodium fluoride on the pineal gland. **What she discovered was quite shocking: the pineal gland simply absorbed more fluoride than any other physical matter in the body, even bones.... fluoride accumulated to strikingly high levels in the pineal gland** and blocks it from functioning properly.

The pineal gland is a sacred part of the human brain; it is the centre of perception and conception. It has the potential to determine the expansion or contraction of our psychic awareness, consciousness, our intuition, *our memory* and *experience with the Divine* but it cannot do it well if it is encrusted with poison. The calcified pineal affects our creativity and intuition and makes us rather docile so that we'll do what we are told to do. (read more in my **'Vibrational Cleaning book**).

Jennifer Luke points out in **another study:** That after half a century of the prophylactic use of fluorides in dentistry, we now know that fluoride readily accumulates in the human pineal gland. In fact, the aged pineal contains more fluoride than any other normal soft tissue.

"Fluoride is likely to cause decreased melatonin production and to have other effects on normal pineal function, which in turn could contribute to a variety of effects in humans." (National Research Council 2006)

Luke's and other studies established that fluoride exposure **contributes to the calcification of the pineal gland.** Upon dissection of a number of pineal glands, the calcification resembled gravel composed of calcite (calcium carbonate) and/or calcium hydroxylapatite. Pineal calcification has been linked with **stroke incidents, schizophrenia, may contribute to melatonin deficiency and circadian timing irregularities, and may be linked to the pathophysiology of tardive dyskinesia and Tourette's syndrome and many other disorders.**

In the 1970's Dr. Dean Burk, a biochemist, co-discoverer of Biotin who was the head chief chemist at the National Cancer Institute – (part of the National Institute of health under the U.S. Department of Health and Human Services) spoke out in an interview in Holland on Fluoride. He stated that adding fluoride to drinking water amounts to public murder on a grand scale. View his interview at https://www.youtube.com/watch?v=ClqK7XvfLg0#t=90 . "Fluoridated Water Is Public Murder on a Grand Scale" – stated Dr. Dean Burk **'It is some of the most conclusive scientific and biological evidence that I have come across in my 50 years in the field of cancer research.'**

IS FLUORIDE REDUCING OUR INTELLIGENCE?

In 2012 Harvard School of Public Health researcher Philippe Grandjean reported that after an extensive amount of research in 42 studies that investigated the relationship between fluoride and human intelligence, 36 of the 42 human studies have found that elevated fluoride exposure is associated with reduced IQ. The human studies, which are based on IQ examinations of over 11,000 children, provide compelling evidence that **fluoride exposure during the early years of life can damage a child's developing brain.**[8] IQ reductions have been significantly associated with fluoride levels of just 0.88 mg/L among children with iodine deficiency.[9] Harvard School of Public Health scientist Philippe Grandjean recently published another revealing study in the March 2014 journal of the Lancet, *classifying fluoride as a neurotoxin. As an esteemed scientist he has classified fluoride in the same category as mercury, arsenic and lead.*

Unfortunately, many children are exposed to fluoride through the oral use of their toothpastes. The 1984 issue of Clinical Toxicology of Commercial Products lists Fluoride as "more poisonous than lead and slightly less poisonous than arsenic". FDA classifies Fluoride as a toxic drug. *So how absurd is it that every morning people are brushing their teeth like good little obedient children- totally brainwashed by the chemical industry to use fluoridated toothpaste?*

Fluoride was added to toothpaste in the mid- 1950's (over 95% of toothpastes today contain Fluoride). It makes people- you - submissive, dutiful and dumb plus it gives you cancer. It poisons and kills you. The only toothpastes without fluoride are the herbal ones that specifically list 'No Fluoride" and one must read the labels carefully. Use the <u>Young Living Thieves</u> essential oil toothpaste which is highly effective and fluoride – chemical free.

So if you want your children to be smarter in school encourage them to use this guaranteed fluoride free – herbal, essential oil toothpaste as well as stopping all fluoridated products and drinking water. Find out more ways to help in eliminating and detoxing fluoride with **'Vibrational Cleaning'** methods.

Pure, authentic, organic, therapeutic, untampered Essential oils have a specific ability to detox these chemicals including Fluoride and activate the pineal !

***—Remember - the EPA has classified these 3 forms of fluoride as toxins: fluorosilicate acid, sodium silicofluoride, and sodium fluoride (used in dentistry)- all are waste products of the nuclear, aluminum and now mostly the phosphate (fertilizer) industries. What are these forms of fluoride doing in our water and toothpaste?

IS FLUORIDE-PROZAC TRAPPING ONE'S SOUL?

Prozac drug (chemical name fluoxetine) is approximately **30% fluoride** by weight and marketed as an "antidepressant,"! Its major side effect, however, from using it or withdrawing from it, is suicidal depression!

Sayer Ji, author /founder of Greenmedinfo points out that Prozac represents a good example of how fluoride affects the personality/soul. The primary reason why Prozac causes a favorable reaction in those who are treated, actually are poisoned with it, is this: the **drug disassociates the person** from the psycho spiritual conflicts that they must normally suppress in order to maintain the appearance of sanity and functionality in society. Modern psychiatry is more about control through drugs and not about true health or healing.

Clear your 3rd eye -pineal from fluoride!

ARE YOU "TRAPPED" TO THE 3RD DIMENSION?

In other words, our pineal is, in part anyway, designed for inter-dimensional access. But when it's calcified, or hardened, it keeps us literally 'locked in' or 'trapped'to this 3rd dimensional reality. You are literally blocked from your **'super powers', your psychic abilities, your intuition** and **your potential as a higher-conscious being of Light**. It's like you are asleep!

For most of us, our pineal gland becomes dormant early in life. This is due to a number of factors which I have pointed out earlier. The on-going chemical pollutants are so pervasive in our lives: found in our food, fluoride & other toxins in our water, our toxic household cleaning agents, dangerous cosmetics and personal care products, poisonous pesticides, insecticides etc. All of these toxins accumulate and calcify the liquid within the pineal gland.

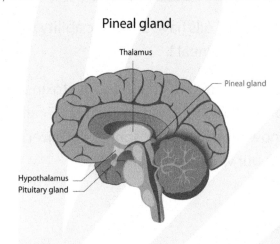

Pineal gland

Thalamus

Pineal gland

Hypothalamus
Pituitary gland

THE VISIBLE ENERGY FIELD - EASILY SHOWS THE PINEAL DISTURBANCE

Science now has a technology to capture energetic information. The Gas Discharge Visualization Technique invented by bio-physicist, visionary, researcher, scientist, Dr. Konstantin Korotkov, advanced a tool for the first time in Science to study the body-mind functions by reading the Human Energy Field. It has been medically approved in Europe with a <u>98% accuracy </u>as a diagnostic tool compared to conventional medical tests.

The Gas Discharge Visualization Kirlian bio-electrography or GDV Kirlian uses cutting-edge camera technology to let the invisible electromagnetic energy field or "aura" that surrounds everything from humans to inanimate objects be seen.

In other words, the camera has allowed for us to capture the energy information about an individual, that is invisible to the eye, but easily seen on the computer screen in real time.

The GDV technique is based on so-called Kirlian effect, named after Semion Kirlian and his wife, who first recorded and studied stimulated electro-photonic images around various objects. GDV studies involve placing the object on a glass electrode into the electric circuit of the device that forms impulses of high-intensity electromagnetic field (with duration 10 micro seconds applied with frequency 1024 Hz). As a result of impulse effect a sequence of gas discharges is formed during the specified exposure time. Spatial distribution of glow emitted by the discharge is registered by the light-sensitive CCD matrix (a charge-coupled device) situated directly under the glass electrode. The obtained image is converted into digital format and recorded on the hard disk of the computer as video files in standard format AVI (Audio Video Interleaved) or in BMP format.

*The GDV camera is the first device in the world which measures the distribution of biological objects. *The Russian Ministry of Health certified the GDV technique as a medical instrument in January 2000.

More developments in the GDV technology have led to the BioWell unit today as a more accessible way to capture the human energy bio-field, better than ever before due to its internet capabilities.

The image, which is created with the Bio-Well instrument, is based on ideas of ***Traditional Chinese Medicine and verified by 18 years of clinical experience*** by hundreds of medical doctors with many thousands of patients. The scanning process is quick, easy and non-intrusive. Visit www.b-wellnow.net

The energy scans have been instrumental over the years for me to track the disturbances in the pineal /pituitary region of the brain.

Below is a bio-field GDV Kirlian picture showing a gap in the head region- an area that is often seen with pituitary/pineal disturbances.

In order to view a bio-field GDV Kirlian picture showing a gap in the head region- an area that is often seen with pituitary/pineal disturbances as well as for more information about this device, visit www.gdv-epckirlian.com.

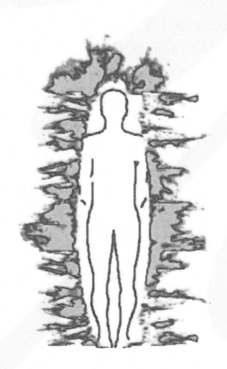

DECALCIFY YOUR PINEAL GLAND
with essential oils

The Pineal Gland is the doorway between the physical and the spiritual. A decalcified pineal will enhance learning, memory, intuition, creativity and maintain youthfulness.

How the essential oils can reach your pineal gland.....

1. **Smell them- Inhale the oil molecules from use in dusting, cleaning, air freshening etc. which will go directly to your pineal.**

2. **Apply directly to the mid- point on your forehead, Crown and the back of the head- the oil will raise your energy system.**

3. **Can add to your water and drink.**

4. **Apply a drop under your tongue for fast absorption into your blood stream.**

5. **Apply a drop on your thumb & touch the roof of your mouth with your thumb. Will absorb directly to the brain.**

(remember these essential oils are live foods and can be eaten at the same time as using them for disinfecting and cleaning)

Essential oils to help decalcify and activate the pineal gland include: Young Living Cedarwood, Brain Power, Lemongrass, Palmarosa, Orange, Sacred Frankincense, Frankincense, Sandalwood, Pine oil, Idaho Blue Spruce, Idaho Balsam Fir and Myrrh.

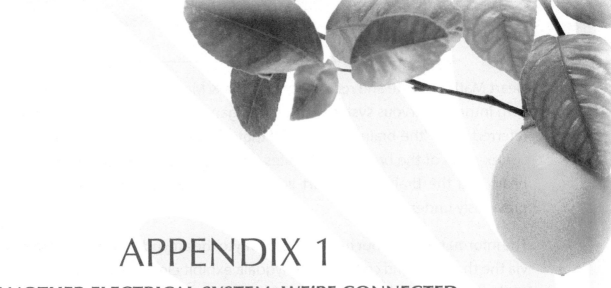

APPENDIX 1
ANOTHER ELECTRICAL SYSTEM: WE'RE CONNECTED
THE HEART – MIND

The heart is not only a pump- it is considered as the 1st brain. It first senses and sends the messages to the brain. The life-force of the human heart is electromagnetic energy that powers the pump. It is also a generator that acts like an oscillating device.

Doctors know that the heart transmits throughout the body a quality and pattern of energy via the heart's electromagnetic field. The Heart Math Institute has been researching and mapping out the patterns of the heart for over thirty years.

The heart communicates with the brain and body in four ways:

Neurological communication (nervous system)

Biophysical communication (pulse wave)

Biochemical communication (hormones)

Energetic communication (electromagnetic fields)

The heart is the most powerful generator of electromagnetic energy in the human body, producing the largest rhythmic electromagnetic field of any of the body's organs. The heart's electrical field is about 60 times greater in amplitude than the electrical activity generated by the brain. This field, measured in the form of an electrocardiogram (ECG), can be detected anywhere on the surface of the body. Furthermore, the magnetic field produced by the heart is more than 5,000 times greater in strength than the field generated by the brain, and can be detected a number of feet away from the body, in all directions, using SQUID-based magnetometers .

Heart Math Institute and researchers Childre & Martin have shown that the heart has its own intrinsic nervous system, with nerve ganglia that processes information, a system referred to as "the brain in the heart' that affects the amygdala, the thalamus and the cortex parts of the brain. This creates a two way communication system between the heart and the brain. The heart is a far more intelligent self-organized system than previously understood.

The information from our heart finds its way to the amygdala, located in the limbic system, via the thalamus and cells in the amygdala exhibit electrical activity that's synchronized to the heart beat. As the heart beat changes, so does the electrical activity change in the cells of the amygdala. There is a direct communication between the heart and the limbic system- specifically the amygdala.

The heart and the brain interconnections are far more important to our states of peace, harmony, love, health and intuition that is based on coherency or incoherency (states of fear, anxiety, anger, depression etc.).

Simply put, coherent people have the power to adapt, thrive mentally, emotionally and physically thus reducing their stress. Researchers at Heart Math have shown that energy drain takes place whether we vent or repress negative mental or emotional states.

In summary, the scientific information now emerging suggest that as people experience sincere positive feeling states, in which the heart's rhythms become more coherent, the changed information flow from the heart to the brain may act to modify cortical function and influence performance. These findings may also help explain the significant shifts in perception, increased mental clarity and heightened intuitive awareness many individuals have reported when practicing the Heart Math techniques. (www.heartmath.org)

Interestingly, the olfactory system is also directly linked to the amygdala- And Emotions are directly linked to the amygdala.

Smells or aromas are processed in the limbic system, considered to be the electrical **emotional** switchboard for the brain bypassing the thalamus. The thalamus is the relay station to and from the cerebral cortex. E.g. like a switchboard which decodes stimuli and sends it to the brain. In other words, one's response to smell is going to be emotional before it can be rational.

The olfactory system has been found to contain 10,000 to 100,000 times more information than sight, taste and touch combined. Olfaction is the only sense that does have a direct effect on the limbic region of the brain. Studies at the University of Vienna have shown that some essential oils and their primary constituents (cineol) can stimulate blood flow and activity in the emotional regions of the brain.

Essential oils have the ability to cross the blood-brain barrier clean and repair as well as stimulate the pineal gland. On a physical level, the Pineal gland is also known to strengthen the thymus (immune system) fight viruses, help to produce antioxidants and rejuvenate the thyroid. With its added functions as a powerful protector against cancer as well as a protector for the heart, having a healthy pineal gland becomes even more obvious to maintain.

The best way that is directly accessible to cleanse and stimulate the Pineal is through smell. (Read Appendix 2 for more information on Emotions & Essential Oils)

When we express love, appreciation or gratitude, we reconnect with the Infinite, the Mind of 'God' and once again our potential becomes limitless. Now with the information in detoxing and activating our pineal glands, we can experience greater depths of our sacredness and our true Divine nature.

We can see, that when we put all this information together, that our olfactory system-aromas, emotions and heart are directly linked to the same part of the brain, the amygdala (our emotional switchboard). With the activation of the pineal, we can see that we have many more possibilities of experiencing the mystical, our spiritual connections along with our physical & emotional balance, making this a truly 'holistic' experience.

"The most beautiful emotion we can experience is the mystical. It is the power of all true art and science. He to whom this emotion is a stranger .. is as good as dead."

-Albert Einstein

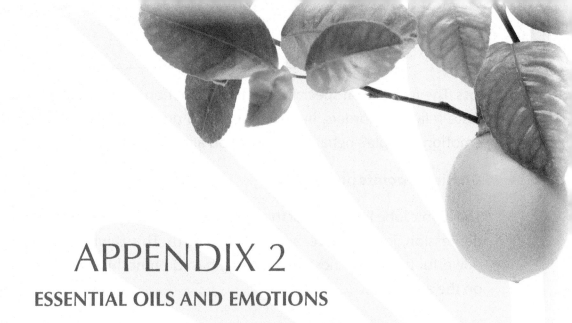

APPENDIX 2
ESSENTIAL OILS AND EMOTIONS

THE POWER OF SMELL

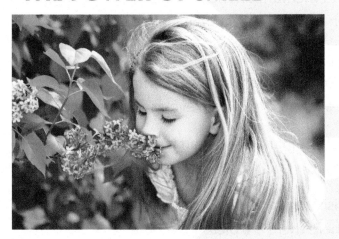

The human olfactory system is our most ancient and powerful root of our emotional life. In other words, the most potent sense is the sense of smell. With its direct access route to the limbic system – particularly to the amygdala, the emotional switchboard of the brain- (as previously mentioned) emotions are triggered quickly.

This is why odors are so strong and memorable- giving them a unique capacity to evoke and transform emotions.

Modern day research has shown that the effects of fragrance and aromatic compounds on the sense of smell exert strong effects on the brain especially on the hypothalamus (the hormone command center of the body) and limbic system (the seat of emotions).

Some essential oils which are high in a particular compound called sesquiterpenes, found in Myrrh, Sandalwood, Cedarwood, Vetiver, Melissa, and Frankincense, can dramatically increase oxygenation and activity in the brain. This may directly improve the function of many systems of the body.

Alan R. Hirsch M.D., F.A.C.P., is the founder and neurologic director of the Smell & Taste Treatment and Independent Research Foundation in Chicago, Illinois. Dr. Hirsch is best known for his extensive research in a variety of documented studies on smell and weight loss. The foundation specializes in the evaluation, diagnosis and treatment of smell and taste-related disorders, including research on how smells and taste can affect human emotion, people's behaviour and mood and disease states.

Dr. Hirsch points out:

The limbic lobe is the part of the brain where we store our emotional memories; anxiety, depression, joy, pleasure, anger and so forth. This is why our sense of smell is such a powerful trigger for nostalgic reverie, based on nothing more than a whiff of an odor on the air.

The understanding that odours evoke more powerful reactions than the other senses do is not a particularly new understanding. It is well known that the aroma of freshly baked goods usually conjures up warm childhood memories. When an odour of baked bread was released in a U.S. supermarket, sales in the bakery section increased threefold.

In summary, the limbic system, the oldest part of the brain, controls emotions, memory and learning, imagination, intuition, and sexuality, as well as the primitive drives and survival instincts. With olfaction any of these can be evoked -- even subconsciously.

Presented below is a summary of some of the remarkable research studies in the area of smell and human behavior:

- One of the studies by Dr. Alan Hirsch discovered that people will judge a product a better value when bought from a shop where there is a pleasant aroma.

- In another study Dr. Hirsch, found that when a mixed floral aroma was suffused throughout a room of calculus students, they increased their speed of learning by 230%.

-The fragrance company Takasago in Japan has shown that data entry errors fell by 20% when lavender was diffused into the atmosphere, reduced by 33% with jasmine and reduced by 54% with lemon. It was also found that by changing the aromas around periodically, workers tolerance to smell and their efficiency could be maintained.

Just a few drops of an essential oil can do wonders - can calm us down, help us to focus, relieve the tensions we all inevitably face. They can relax our muscles, improve our digestion, and help us get a fantastic night's sleep or remember what we need to remember. They can also help **to release deep held memories and emotions.**

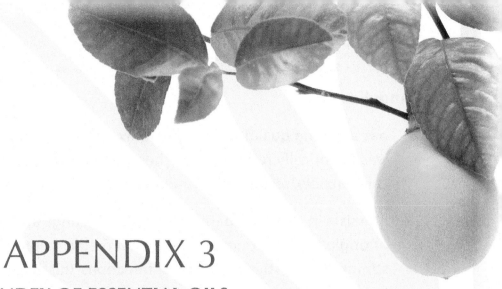

APPENDIX 3
INDEX OF ESSENTIAL OILS

SPECIFIC ESSENTIAL OILS FOR THE PINEAL WHILE YOU ARE "GREENERIZING" YOUR CLEANING
GREEN CLEAN AND CLEAN YOUR PINEAL TOO

The Essential oils are listed below to specifically green clean and stimulate the Pineal, Pituitary glands at the same time. These alternative essential oil cleansers will help you tremendously to detox and activate the Pineal gland while cleaning, sanitizing, disinfecting or using them as an air freshener in your home/office: All the various ways outlined in the above chapters for cleaning, sanitizing, washing will aid in your enjoyment of these treasured gifts from nature.

Lemon:

Via its vapors alone will help to cleanse your pineal by digesting hydrocarbon deposits that block or cloud this gland.

- **Home Uses:** Use in your dishwasher and enjoy the fresh, lemony smell.

- Add to you baking soda for scrubs and washing counter tops, tubs and many other tips already presented earlier in this book.

- Diffuse to freshen your home or add a few drops to a spray bottle to deodorize and sterilize the air.

- Add ten drops to a cotton ball and place inside your vacuum cleaner- see the many other ways in the earlier chapter

Angelica :

- has soothing qualities that help relax nerves and muscles. In Germany, angelica was historically referred to as the "oil of angels," in part because of its ability to calm anxiety, restore happy memories, and bring peaceful sleep.

- It assists in releasing pent-up negative feelings and restores memories to point of origin prior to traumas. Traditional medicine practitioners used angelica as a stimulant, digestive tonic, aid for infections, (historically it was credited to protect from the plague) and expectorant.

  Home Uses: Use in your dishwasher and enjoy the smell.

- Add to your potpourris as an air freshener

- Diffuse to freshen your home or add a few drops to a spray bottle to deodorize and sterilize the air.

Orange:

Via its vapors helps to digest petrochemicals esp. in the brain.

- **Home Uses:** Disinfectant for toilets, laundry room, kitchen,

- Mix in a spray bottle to disinfect fruit/vegetables

- Use for Countertops/cutting boards

- Sterilizes surfaces, kills microbes, disinfectant

- Add to your dishwasher

116

Cedarwood:

- (Cedrus atlantica) – has a woodsy, warm, balsamic aroma. It is very high in sesquiterpenes.

- Its powerful scent creates a relaxing, calming and comforting atmosphere when diffused.

- Cedarwood essential oil has many purifying properties along with its known fungicidal properties.

- Cedarwood (Cedrus atlantica) essential oil can be added to your favorite skin care products and applied topically.

Vetiver:

Vetiver Essential Oil is very grounding and the aroma is very earthy.

- Vetiver oil is psychologically grounding, calming, relaxing and stabilizing.

- One of the oils that is highest in sesquiterpenes, vetiver was studied by Dr. Terry Friedmann for improving children's behavior.

- Vetiver may help when coping with stress and to recover from emotional trauma and shock. Emotionally grounding.

- Supports restful sleep and supports a healthy, normal circulatory system

- Has rejuvenating qualities for mature skin, especially sagging skin

- Home Uses: Use as a deodorizer by adding 10 drops to a spray bottle or to a diffuser.

- Helps to cope with stress and recover from emotional trauma- mix a few drops in oil/vinegar mixture to make your furniture polish.

Lemongrass:

Powerful, easy, versatile essential oil.

- Lemongrass (Cymbopogon flexuosus) essential oil supports overall well-being and may support the digestive system. This oil contains the naturally occurring constituent geranial.

- Great support for healthy joints, ligaments, tendons and cartilage function

- Helpful in keeping unwanted insects at bay.

- Supports connective tissue function

- Used traditionally as a flavor enhancer by many cultures, adding Lemongrass oil is a delightful way to enhance the flavor of meals. It also helps to support normal digestion.

- Helps to balance the parasympathetic nervous system,

- Supports deep overall cleansing

- Lemongrass also protects our auric field from electromagnetic energy (TV, computers, radio).

***Can cause extreme skin irritation therefore, dilution is highly recommended if applied to the skin.

- Home Uses: Since it is helpful for bacterial- salmonella issues- use for cleaning countertops, sinks, refrigerators, stove tops and any kitchen surface.

- Helps to promote psychic awareness and purification- use in your diffuser or as an air freshener and for cleaning any surface area.

Palmarosa:

- Home Uses: Use in scouring powder – Add 20 drops of Palmarosa to 1 cup of baking soda.

- Apply to laundry wash - 10 -15 drops to a laundry load.

- Wash kitchen countertops with cloth soaked with Palmarosa

- Spritz cutting boards with water mixed with Palmarosa

- Deodorize your refrigerator.

- Palmarosa has recently been found in numerous studies to be a neuro-protective

Sandalwood:

- Sandalwood Essential Oil is high in sesquiterpenes the chemical component that stimulates the pineal gland in the brain.

- Helps to oxygenate the pineal/pituitary glands improving frequency balance

- Creates deep relaxation of the nervous system and that is why it has been used for centuries to enhance meditation.

- Used traditionally as incense in religious ceremonies and for meditation, this oil is uplifting and relaxing.

- Fragrance helps to remove negative programming from the cells, stimulating for the pineal gland.

- It is valued in skin care for its moisturizing and normalizing properties.

- Home Uses: Use as a deodorizer.

- Diffuse in the room for relaxation and /or meditation.

- Add several drops to a spray bottle with water and spritz bed sheets.

Helichrysum:

- Helichrysum (Helichrysum italicum) is known for its restorative properties and provides excellent support to the skin, liver and nervous system.

- Scores high on the ORAC scale an amazing 17,430.

- Helichrysum also provides a defense against harmful free radicals, making it a vital ingredient in several Young Living blends.

- It has the properties to detox fluoride and petrochemicals from the Pineal helping to bring balance and harmony to the glandular system.

- The fragrance is uplifting to the subconscious.

- Helichrysum essential oil is a fantastic support for the circulatory system. It possesses regenerative properties that make it fantastic for supporting and maintaining any skin condition. It is even considered to be a natural helper for skin care from the sun!

- Use For: Circulatory Support, Muscle Tension, Restorative Properties.

- Home Uses: Add 2-3 drops to a spray bottle with water and spritz bed sheets.

- Use in your bath water- mix 2-3 drops with sea salt or Epsom salts.

- Create a salt rub- add 3 drops to ½ cup sea salt withy 2 tbsp of almond oil – rub a small handful over skin while showering.

- Mix 3-6 drops with 100 drops of sesame oil or olive oil as your natural skin care in the sun.

Idaho Balsam Fir:

- Traditionally used for muscular aches and pains, and for fever, rheumatic pain and any kind of respiratory function, this herbaceous oil can be diffused for aromatherapy or diluted with carrier oil for topical application.

- The warm aroma of balsam fir soothes and rejuvenates the body and mind.

- It is also believed to create an uplifting sense of well-being.

- Helps to regenerate telomeres to their normal, healthy function, to reduce stress by helping to reduce cortisol-stress hormone production and restore calmness to the body-mind

- Balsam Fir oil is also very soothing for muscles (or joints and tendons) that have been overworked or are tired.

- Home Uses: Add drops to a spray bottle and spritz linen, wardrobe, drawers.

- Use as a potpourri or deodorizer.

- Add drops to a cotton ball and place in drawers.

- Be creative in adding it into your daily routines.

Sacred Frankincense:

- Rarest, most sought-after aromatic in existence.

- The frankincense of the ancients and the traditional spiritual oil of biblical times.

- Contains incensole acetate- the molecule or constituent for spiritual awareness

- Primary Benefits

- Deepens spiritual connection.

- Supplements Boswellia carteri's everyday application.

- Diffuse in your homes- use the resin as well for air purification.

Xiang Mao:

Was discovered high in Taiwan's southeastern mountain slopes. It is ccommonly known as red lemongrass. Xiang Mao means "aromatic grass for rapid enlightenment" and is a rapid-growing clump grass that can grow up to 6 feet tall.

Xiang Mao was traditionally used to freshen household air, enlighten the mind, and moisturize skin. It was also used in folk medicine for its calming effects and to promote relaxation. Xiang Mao's benefits and versatility make it ideal for many everyday home and personal uses.

Home Uses:

- **Diffuse Xiang Mao alone or with Citronella, Cedarwood, Patchouli or Myrtle to create a natural, potent pesticide-free, safe insect deterrent.**

- **Use the above-mentioned oils to create a natural bug spray. Use 10–20 drops of each oil in a base of distilled water or drop the oils into standing water around your yard and home to help prevent mosquitoes.**

- **Use this oil as a cleansing agent to help purify surfaces. Add it to Thieves® Household Cleaner. Can also add 20–30 drops in a small spray bottle of distilled water and use it on countertops.**

- **For furniture polish, add 20-30 drops to ½ cup olive oil to protect and nourish wood furniture.**

- **Use Xiang Mao in your diffuser or as an air freshener by adding drops to cotton balls and leave in drawers of linen closet.**

- **Make an all-natural soap with this new single oil.**

Unique Pine Essential Oil:

Has a long history of uses since the time of Hippocrates. The Native Americans used pine needles in bedding by stuffing them in mattresses to repel bedbugs, lice and fleas. It was used to treat lung infections and is similar to many of the healing and disinfecting properties of Eucalyptus globulus essential oil.

Pine oil's powerful capacities are due to its high levels of phenols, the acidic plant chemicals that fight off germs and ward off disease. At the same time, pine essential oil has the ability to reduce inflammation and associated redness, aid the body in cleansing impurities, fight off sinus infections, clear mucus and phlegm, cure skin conditions like eczema and psoriasis*, boost your immune system, fight fungal and viral infections (great for colds and flues), relieve anxiety (anxiolytic effect) and revitalize the mind, body and spirit, plus protect your home and body from a wide variety of germs.

Pine oil has also been used to improve eye health, (e.g. macular degeneration, cataracts), reduce inflammation of the gall bladder, asthma, catarrh, coughs, laryngitis, Urinary Tract Infections (UTI), excellent mood elevator (http://www.ncbi.nlm.nih.gov/pmc/articles/PMC3173901) and stress reducer, as well as its use for weakened concentration and memory loss.

*Dermatologists often prescribe the oil for treating psoriasis, itching, pimples, eczema, skin diseases, poor skin, scabies, sores, and fleas. Frequent use helps to keep the skin smooth, renewed and shiny and also acts as an antioxidant for free radicals.

Pine (Pinus sylvestris) has a refreshing, invigorating aroma. Due to its numerous health benefits and varied widespread uses, the pine essential oil has become one of the most important essential oils used in aromatherapy today.

Word of Caution:

Avoid any pine essential oils adulterated with turpentine, low-cost, but potentially hazardous filler. Hence the reason it is most important to know your company - I strongly recommend to only use food-therapeutic grade Young Living essential oils.

- **Home Uses: Always use food grade pine oil!**

- **Use as a floor cleaner: mix ½ cup white vinegar, several drops of pine essential oil into a bucket of warm water. Ready to mop away.**

- **Disinfect kitchen sinks, countertops as well as bathrooms: simply mix 5-6 drops of pine oil in an 8 oz spray bottle. Spray over the area and wipe clean.**

- **Add several drops to your household detergent such as the Thieves cleaner to further disinfect a sick room**

- **Great for vapor therapy in a sick room as it promotes healing for sinuses and respiratory conditions. Add several drops to your steamer or vaporizer.**

- **Flavor enhancer to foods: Add to your beverages - dilute one drop in 4 fl. oz. of**

liquid such as goat's, coconut or rice milk. Add a drop to flavor baked goods or puddings

- **Use in closets to protect your wool sweaters from moths and other insects. Drop 8-10 drops of Pine essential oil onto pieces of dried wood to place in your closets or drawers. Can apply several drops of pine oil on pine cones that can hang in your closet.**

- **Delight your senses and mood by adding 4-6 drops of pine essential oil to a spray bottle to spray the room to rid stale or toxic air. Just avoid spraying it on furniture.**

- **Create your own massage blend as pine is soothing for stressed muscles and joints when used in massage. Add 3-5 drops of pine essential oil to 2 ounces of almond or jojoba oil.**

- **Add 1-2 drops of Pine essential oil to ½ cup olive oil and mix in a bowl- Use a damp cloth to dip and use for dusting furniture.**

Possible skin sensitivity. If pregnant or under a doctor's care, consult your physician. Do not use near fire, flame, heat or spark. Dilution recommended for both topical and internal use.

More Interesting Data on the Pine Oil – Perfect for YOUR THIRD EYE

This oil becomes a very extraordinary oil to use for many special reasons as listed above but also because of what it can do to support and maintain a healthy, highly-functioning pineal gland. (Pine is high in alpha-pinene which has been shown to have an anxiolytic effect- see study below *).

The pine cone itself is the common symbol found in many ancient cultures widely depicted in Egyptian symbolism associated with enlightenment and an opening to greater spiritual dimensions through the pineal gland. (The pine cone symbol is used on the front cover of the Vibrational Cleaning book). Both the pineal gland and the pine cone have a similar shape.

Images of the pine cone used on the staff of Osiris, and the staff held by the pope as well as in the Vatican court yard, for instance, show a rising of energy (the staff) followed by the opening "petals" of the pine cone at the peak. This representation signifies the enlightenment experience where the pineal gland produces unique secretions of substances like DMT (discussed in the "Vibrational Cleaning" book) and other neurotransmitters that unlock higher awareness.

Another product worth mentioning and quite intriguing is the Pine pollen powder. The nuts (from the female cones) and the inner bark have both been used as a food as well as medicine by traditional cultures. Pine pollen powder has been used extensively in traditional cultures throughout Asia. The earliest mention of pine tree pollen's medicinal use is in Chinese herbalism.

*Anxiolytic (relieving anxiety) effect. (http://www.ncbi.nlm.nih.gov/pubmed/25340185)

*Alpha-pinene has been known to possess anti-inflammatory properties which may be beneficial to alleviate neurodegenerative diseases including Alzheimer's and Parkinson's. In one study, the researchers found alpha-pinene to decrease the inflammatory markers concluding that alpha-pinene may be an alternative ant-inflammatory agent to prevent and/or cure the neurodegenerative diseases. (http://herbalnet.healthrepository.org/handle/123456789/2619)

Brain Power:

- **Assists with mental clarity and helps to support normal, healthy brain function.**

- **Increases oxygen around the pineal, pituitary and hypothalamus of the brain.**

- **It is known to help cleanse petrochemicals around the glands in the brain and along the spine when used in massage that supports brain health.**

- **Stimulates the pineal gland responsible to metabolize 50% serotonin in the body.**

- **Brain Power™ gives your brain a boost with essential oils that are high in sesquiterpenes. Use it to clarify thought and develop greater focus.**

- **Home Uses: use as an air freshener, add to spritzer bottles to spray sheets and your clothing.**

- **Add a few drops to a cotton ball and place in your drawers.**

- Add to a damp cloth for your laundry.

- Add to sea salt or Epsom salts for bathing:

- Spritz your face with a mixture of 2-3 drops with water in a spray bottle daily.

Awaken:

- Awaken™ is an inspiring combination of several essential oil blends that helps bring about inner awareness and awakening, helping to strengthen the desire to reach one's potential. True understanding of one's self is the first step toward making successful changes and desirable transitions. This blend may help you progress toward your highest potential.

- Awaken will amplify the function of the pineal and pituitary glands and help stimulate the creativity and intuitive side of the right brain. Feeling stuck in the left logical side of your brain? Then you'll want to increase your spiritual awareness, with the Awaken Essential Oil blend.

- Home Uses:

- Use in your dishwasher and enjoy the smell.

- Add to your potpourris as an air freshener

- Diffuse to freshen your home or office by adding a few drops to a spray bottle to deodorize and sterilize the air.

Inspiration:

Inspiration™ includes oils of sandalwood, frankincense, cedarwood, rosewood, myrtle, spruce and mugwort traditionally used for hundreds of years by the native peoples of Arabia, India, and North America for enhancing spirituality, prayer, meditation and inner awareness.

It creates an aromatic sanctuary for those seeking quiet meditation and spirituality. This specific blend helps to find a calm space in our minds helping to release negative thoughts that can block our connection with the divine. Inspiration helps to enhance the pituitary and pineal glands of the body.

Home Uses: use as an air freshener, add to spritzer bottles to spray sheets and your clothing

- **Add a few drops to a cotton ball and place in your drawers**

- **Add to a damp cloth for your laundry**

- **Add to sea salt or Epsom salts for bathing:**

- **Add to dried flowers to create a potpourri**

- **Add to your diffuser to imbue the space**

Into The Future:

- This essential Oil blend is an excellent aid for moving forward into the future and leaving the past behind. Into the Future™ was formulated to foster feelings of determination and a pioneering spirit, helping you leave the past behind so that you can move forward. This uplifting oil also helps with visualization and meditation.

- Using this blend will enhance enjoyment of challenges leading to success and help to overcome fear of the unknown.

- **Home Uses: use as an air freshener, add to spritzer bottles to spray sheets and your clothing**

- **Add a few drops to a cotton ball and place in your drawers**

- **Add to a damp cloth for your laundry.**

- **Add to sea salt or Epsom salts for bathing.**

- **Add to dried flowers to create a potpourri.**

- **Add to your diffuser to imbue the space.**

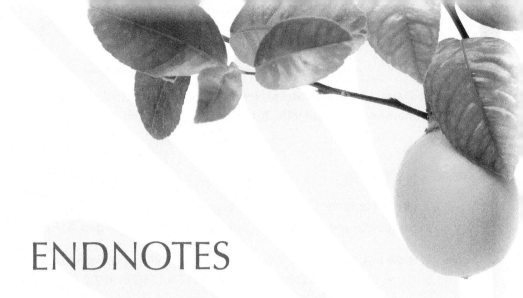

ENDNOTES

SOURCES:

CHAPTER 1

1. CDC- **http://www.cdc.gov/nczved/divisions/dfbmd/diseases/campylobacter/**

2. Food Control 18 (2007) 414–420

www.elsevier.com/locate/foodcont

Inhibitory eVects of selected plant essential oils on the growth of four

pathogenic bacteria: E. coli O157:H7, Salmonella Typhimurium,

Staphylococcus aureus and Listeria monocytogenes

Mounia Oussalah, Stéphane Caillet, Linda Saucier, Monique Lacroix.

3. Antimicrobial activity of five essential oils against origin strains of the Enterobacteriaceae family.

Penalver P, Huerta B, Borge C, et al. Antimicrobial activity of five essential oils against origin strains of the Enterobacteriaceae famly. APMIS. 2005;113:1-6.

4. Science Daily, 'Essential Oils May Provide Good Source of Food Preservation'

http://www.sciencedaily.com/releases/2014/07/140718114545.htm

5. Caio G. Otoni, Silvania F. O. Pontes, Eber A. A. Medeiros, Nilda de F. F. Soares. **Edible Films from Methylcellulose and Nanoemulsions of Clove Bud (Syzygium aromaticum) and Oregano (Origanum vulgare) Essential Oils as Shelf Life Extenders for Sliced Bread**. *Journal of Agricultural and Food Chemistry*, 2014; 62 (22): 5214 DOI: 10.1021/jf501055f

6. J Appl Microbiol. 2006 Dec;101(6):1232-40.

The effect of lemon, orange and bergamot essential oils and their components on the survival of Campylobacter jejuni, Escherichia coli O157, Listeria monocytogenes, Bacillus cereus and Staphylococcus aureus in vitro and in food systems.

Fisher K[1], Phillips CA.

7. **David** Gutierrez, **Natural News Aug. 02, 2014 http://www.naturalnews.com/046287_cinnamon_essential_oils_foodborne_illness.html**

CHAPTER 2

1. Cheryl Luptowski, home-safety expert and public information officer, NSF International (a global public health and safety organization), Ann Arbor, Michigan. NSF.org

2. Desai MA, et al. Reduction of Listeria monocytogenes Biofilms on Stainless Steel and Polystyrene Surfaces by Essential Oils, J Food Prot. 2012 Jul;75(7):1332-7.

3. "Antibiotics in food and animals and facts about meat labels," April 9, 2013. http://paleochik.com/2013/04/09/antibiotics-in-food-animals-and-facts-about-meat-labels/.

4. Venkitanarayanan K, et al., "Use of plant-derived antimicrobials for improving the safety of poultry products," *Poult Sci.* 2013 Feb;92(2):493-501.

5. *Essential Oil Desk Reference, Fifth Edition*. Life Science Publishing, 2011

CHAPTER 3

1. CDC **(http://www.cdc.gov/drugresistance/threat-report-2013/**

2.(http://www.dailymail.co.uk/health/article-157079/What-truth-MRSA-superbug.html#ixzz39yK8s8jj)

3.**http://www.educationpost.com.hk/resources/healthcare/140505-healthcare-news-one-new-superbug-infection-every-18-minutes-hong-kong-public**

4.Liz Szabo, "CDC sounds alarm on deadly, untreatable super bugs," USA Today, March 6, 2013, http://www.usatoday.com/story/news/nation/2013/03/05/superbugs-infections-hospitals/1965133/.

5. Bachir RG, Benali M, "Antibacterial activity of the essential oils from the leaves of *Eucalyptus globulus* against *Escherichia coli* and *Staphylococcus aureus*," *Asian Pac J. Trop Biomed.* 2012 Sep;2(9):739-42.

6. Laird K, et al. Reduction of surface contamination and biofilms of Enterococcus sp. and Staphylococcus aureus using a citrus-based vapour, J Hosp Infect. 2012 Kam'80(1):61-6.

7. Science Daily, 'Essential oils to fight superbugs' http://www.sciencedaily.com/releases/2010/03/100330210942.htm

CHAPTER 4

No Endnotes

CHAPTER 5

1. *Essential Oil Desk Reference, Fifth Edition*. Life Science Publishing, 2011

2. US EPA, http://www.epa.gov

3. Close, Edward, http://moldrx4u.com

4. Pendleton SJ, et al., "Inhibition of beef isolates of E. coli 0157:H7 by orange oil at various temperatures," J Food Sci. 2012 Jun;77(6):M308-11.

5. Michiels J, "Effect of organic acids on Salmonella colonization and shedding in weaned piglets in a seeder model," J Food Prot. 2012 Nov;75(11):1974-83.

6. Simitzis PE, et al., "Effect of dietary oregano oil supplementation on lamb meat characteristics," Meat Sci. 2008 Jun;79(2):217-23.

7. Lu Y, Wu C, "Reduction of Salmonella enterica contamination on grape tomatoes by washing with thyme oil, thymol, and carvacrol as compared with chlorine treatment," J Food Prot. 2010 Dec;73(12):2270-5.

8. Muriel-Galet V, et al., "Development of antimicrobial films for microbiological control of packaged salads," Int. J Food Microbiol. 2012 Jul 2;157(2):195-201.

CHAPTER 6

No Endnotes

CHAPTER 7

1. Mercola, (http://articles.mercola.com/sites/articles/archive/2014/08/23/mosquito-repellent.aspx?e_cid=20140823Z1_PRNL_art_1&utm_source=prmrnl&utm_medium=email&utm_content=art1&utm_campaign=20140823Z1&et_cid=DM54227&et_rid=632335865)

2. Zhang QH, et al., "Essential oils and their compositions as spatial repellents for pestiferous wasps," *Pest Manag Sci.* 2012 Aug 28.

3. Oussalah, M. "Antimicrobial and Antioxidant Effects of Milk Protein-Based Film Containing Essential Oils for the Preservation of Whole Beef Muscle." *J Agric Food Chem*. 52. no. 18 (2004): 5598-5605. http://pubs.acs.org/doi/abs/10.1021/jf049389q (accessed April 8, 2013).

4. Oussalah, M. "Antimicrobial effects of selected plant essential oils on the growth of a Pseudomonas putida strain isolated from meat." *Meat Science*. 73. no. 2 (2006): 236-244. http://www.ncbi.nlm.nih.gov/pubmed/22062294 (accessed April 8, 2013).

5. Huff, Ethan A. "The best, and worst, laundry detergents with 1,4 dioxane contamination." *Natural News*, May 22, 2010. http://www.naturalnews.com/028846_laundry_detergents_dioxane.html

6. Exley, C. "Aluminium in human breast tissue.." *Journal of Inorganic Chemistry*. 101. no. 9 (2007): 1344-1346. http://www.ncbi.nlm.nih.gov/pubmed/17629949 (accessed March 29, 2013).

7. Mercola, Joseph. "99 percent of Breast Cancer Tissue Contained This Everyday Chemical (NOT Aluminum)." May 24, 2012. http://articles.mercola.com/sites/articles/archive/2012/05/24/parabens-on-risk-of-breast-cancer.aspx (accessed March 29, 2013).

8. Main, Emily. "How to Stay Bug Free without Dangerous DEET." *Rodale*, . http://www.rodale.com/mosquito-repellants-without-deet (accessed April 9, 2013).

9. Abou-Donia, MB. "Co-exposure to pyridostigmine bromide, DEET, and/or permethrin causes sensorimotor deficit and alterations in brain acetylcholinesterase activity." *Pharmacol Biochem Behav*. no. 2 (2004): 253-262. http://www.ncbi.nlm.nih.gov/pubmed/14751452 (accessed April 9, 2013).

10. US EPA, "Permethrin Facts (RED Fact Sheet)." Accessed April 9, 2013. http://www.epa.gov/oppsrrd1/REDs/factsheets/permethrin_fs.htm.

11. Environmental Health, "Hazards of DEET." Last modified 2003. Accessed April 9, 2013. http://www.environmentalhealth.ca/spring03hazards.html.

12. Stanczyk, Nina. "Aedes aegypti Mosquitoes Exhibit Decreased Repellency by DEET following Previous Exposure." *PLOS One*. (2013). http://www.plosone.org/article/info:doi/10.1371/journal.pone.0054438 (accessed April 9, 2013).

13. Qualls, WA. "Field evaluation of commercial repellents against the floodwater mosquito Psorophora columbiae (Diptera: Culicidae) in St. Johns County, Florida." *Journal of Medical Entomology*. no. 6 (2011): 1247-1249. http://www.ncbi.nlm.nih.gov/pubmed/22238886 (accessed April 9, 2013).

14. Centers for Disease Control and Prevention, "Insect Repellent Use and Safety." Accessed April 9, 2013. http://www.cdc.gov/ncidod/dvbid/westnile/qa/insect_repellent.htm.

15. Gabriel, Julie. *The Green Beauty Guide: Your Essential Resource to Organic and Natural Skin Care, Hair Care, Makeup, and Fragrances*. HCI, 2008.

16. Mercola, Joseph. "Cinnamon Oil Better for Killing Mosquitoes Than DEET." *Mercola.com*, August 07, 2004. http://articles.mercola.com/sites/articles/archive/2004/08/07/cinnamon-oil-deet.aspx (accessed April 9, 2013).

CHAPTER 8

1. Connett, Michael. "Fluoride & Intelligence: The 36 Studies." *Fluoride Action Network*, December 09, 2012. http://www.fluoridealert.org/studies/brain01/ (accessed April 8, 2013).

2. Connett, Michael. "The Facts About Fluoride & Human Intelligence." *Waking Times*, November 03, 2012. http://www.wakingtimes.com/2012/11/03/the-facts-about-fluoride-human-intelligence/ (accessed April 8, 2013).

ABOUT THE AUTHOR

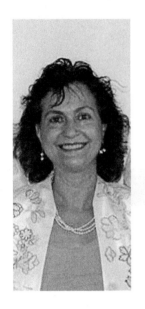

Sabina M. DeVita (Ed.D, D.N.M. N.N.C.P., IASP, CBP, DCSJ) has been a long time environmentalist. When she became ill in the 1980's, with environmental sensitivities, also known as ecological illness or multiple chemical sensitivities (MCS), she was **forced to change her life path dramatically.** She experienced many ill effects physically, mentally and emotionally from environmental and **chemical sensitivities**.

She left her position as a teacher then guidance counsellor of many years in the public school system to pursue her doctoral interests in psychology and environmental sensitivities due to her illness. Her doctoral dissertation on **brain allergies** and mental health issues, a rare combination not at all known or considered even to this day, became **the first work of its kind** in the field of psychology at the University of Toronto as well as in environmental & ecological sensitivities.

In the late 90's she discovered the power of real, organic, therapeutic grade A essential oils and the art & science of **French medicinal aromatherapy**. She became involved with the company that is the World Leader in Essential oils, the "Seed to Seal" Young Living company. These precious and live-food essential oils were introduced into her practices and in all of her classes as a powerful solution to many of human kinds' ills along with her energy dowsing and kinesiology techniques.

She is certified as a Registered Nutritional coach-consultant and Doctor in Natural Medicine as well as in Holistic Energy Psychology and Essential oils sciences, Egyptian dowsing and specialized Kinesiology and Body Talk. She is Director and Founder of the DeVita Wellness Institute of Living and Learning with 27 years as an eclectic psychotherapist. She is also Director – Founder of the federally approved Institute of

131

Energy Wellness Studies of the last 7 years. Dr. DeVita is an accomplished author of five books and an international speaker. She was trained by D. Gary Young founder of Young Living Essential Oils with over 850 hours in essential oil sciences and application and certified by him in 2007 as a Raindrop technique Instructor.

Dr. DeVita is certified in Russia as a GDV Kirlian Bio-electrographic practitioner and instructor by the inventor scientist, physicist, Dr. K. Korotkov. She holds Grand master in Belvaspata. She is a graduate from the Bio-Geometry program on the **physics of quality** with both Dr. Robert Gilbert and Dr. Ibrahim Karim (founder of Bio-Geometry) and incorporates some of the simple Bio- Geometry principles in her teachings and writings.

CPSIA information can be obtained at www.ICGtesting.com
Printed in the USA
LVOW02s1321140815

450153LV00011B/173/P